# Simplicity

## Creating Physical, Mental, and Emotional Health Awareness

Gord Lund

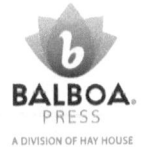

**BALBOA.**
PRESS

A DIVISION OF HAY HOUSE

Balboa Press books may be ordered through booksellers or by contacting:

Balboa Press
A Division of Hay House
1663 Liberty Drive
Bloomington, IN 47403
www.balboapress.com
1-(877) 407-4847

Because of the dynamic nature of the Internet, any web addresses or links contained in this book may have changed since publication and may no longer be valid. The views expressed in this work are solely those of the author and do not necessarily reflect the views of the publisher, and the publisher hereby disclaims any responsibility for them.

The author of this book does not dispense medical advice or prescribe the use of any technique as a form of treatment for physical, emotional, or medical problems without the advice of a physician, either directly or indirectly. The intent of the author is only to offer information of a general nature to help you in your quest for emotional and spiritual well-being. In the event you use any of the information in this book for yourself, which is your constitutional right, the author and the publisher assume no responsibility for your actions.

Any people depicted in stock imagery provided by Thinkstock are models, and such images are being used for illustrative purposes only. Certain stock imagery © Thinkstock.

ISBN: 978-1-4525-6227-8 (sc)
ISBN: 978-1-4525-6228-5 (e)

Printed in the United States of America

Balboa Press rev. date: 11/19/2012

# Index

# PREFACE

This book was created while trekking in the Himalayas.

The reason for writing this book is to create physical, mental and emotional health awareness in a simple, powerful format.

Because we live in an environment of misinformation we need to be educated and take a preventative approach to our health and wellness.

"Believe nothing, no matter where you read it, or who said it, even if I have said it, unless it agrees with your own reason and common sense."

Buddha

Goals for reading this book:

Adding 1 – 2 or 3 things to our lifestyle and diet.

Eliminating 1 – 2 or 3 things from our lifestyle and diet.

"Health is the real wealth, not pieces of gold and silver"

Ghandi

Information in this book is in alignment with my personal opinions, knowledge, beliefs, values and wisdom.

Gord Lund

# FORWARD

There are two choices in our lives regarding health.

We are either making life affirming choices or we are making choices that compromise our well being.

What we choose either helps us grow, live and bring life and light into our bodies and experience or we choose darkness, decay, ill health and death.

There are many golden gems in this book that have the potential to plant seeds for lifelong transformations.

Seeds of possibility that with the wisdom contained in this book nourish the fertile soil of the human body mind temple.

Gord is a man who lives and teaches simplicity in a time where it is greatly needed, if we are willing to be open and receptive to its rays.

In this simplistic platform, readers have the opportunity to be exposed to the information that provides breakthroughs in emotional, physical and mental health well being.

Gord is a genius of simplicity and inspires those who come into contact with his presence, words and gems of wisdom.

In love, light and infinite gratitude.

Jaime Onofrey

ReelEyes Productions Conscious Media

# SIMPLISTIC QUOTES

Thomas Mattiessen
" Life is beautiful in its simplicity."

Issac Newton
"Nature is pleased with simplicity."

Leonardo da Vinci
"Simplicity is the ultimate sophistication."

Norman Vincent Peale
"We struggle with complexities and avoid the simplicities."

Confucius
"Life is really simple, but we insist on making it complicated."

John C. Maxwell
"Educators take something simple and make it complicated
communicators take something complicated and make it simple."

Albert Einstein
"God always takes the simplest way."

Albert Einstein
"If you can't explain it simply, you don't understand it well enough."

Winston Churchill
"A vocabulary of truth and simplicity will be of service throughout your life."

Plato
"Beauty of style and harmony and grace and good rhythm depend on simplicity."

Charles Mingus
"Making the simple complicated is commonplace; making the complicate simple, awesomely simple, that's creativity."

Ronald Reagan
"They say the world has become too complicated for simple answers, they are wrong."

Leo Tzui
"I have three things to teach: simplicity, patience, compassion, these three are your greatest treasure."

Henry Wadsworth Longfellow
"In character, in style, in all things, the supreme excellence is simplicity."

Leo Nikolaevich Tolstov
"There is no greatness where there is not simplicity, goodness and truth."

George Earle Buckle
"To simplify complications is the first essential of success."

# CAUSES of DEATH

Figures below show us how important it is to personally take control of our health.

Heart disease – 28%

Cancer – 25%

Medical Drugs – 8%

Infections in Hospitals – 7%

Stroke – 6%

Lower Respiratory – 6%

Iatrogenic – 4% medical errors causing death by Doctors.

Alzheimer's – 4%

Diabetes – 4%

Pneumonia / Influenza – 3%

Nephritis – Kidney – 2%

Septicemia – Blood Bacteria – 1%

HIV – Aids – 1%

Liver Disease – 1%

    National Center for Health Statistics – Time Magazine

Medical Drugs – causing 8% of deaths represent only deaths that are reported.

Infections in Hospitals – causing 6% of deaths represent only deaths that are reported.

Iatrogenic Errors - causing 4% of deaths represent only deaths that are reported.

90% of surgeries and procedures are considered unnecessary.

90% of prescription drugs are considered unnecessary.

# DRUG TOXICITY

Medical drugs – create a state of mental and physical imbalances in the body.

More people today get:

Flu's

Colds

Cancer

Diabetes

Heart Disease

Asthma

More people today are taking:

Prescription Drugs

Non Prescription Drugs

Most drugs merely postpone disease eruptions, which are likely to occur in the future.

1/3 of people are admitted to hospital because of toxic side effects of medications.

It is estimated that 45,000 people die each year in North America from the use of over the counter pain killers like aspirin, plus painkiller drugs cause widespread stomach ulcers.

All over the counter drugs carry the risk of hazardous side effects, especially those under these categories:

| | |
|---|---|
| pain killers | indigestion |
| heartburn | cold medicines |
| anti inflammatory | cough medicines |

90% of the patients who visit doctors have conditions that will either improve on their own or that are out of the reach of modern medicines ability to solve.

Below are examples of potential drug side effects:

Amoxicillin – a penicillin antibiotic – fights bacteria in your body:

| | |
|---|---|
| seizures – fever | confusion |
| dark urine | severe diarrhea |
| cloudy stools | difficulty breathing |

OxyContin – is a narcotic pain killer:

| | |
|---|---|
| convulsions | headache |
| constipation | slow heartbeat |
| nausea – vomiting | shallow breathing |

Lipitor – statin drug – used to treat high cholesterol:

| | |
|---|---|
| vomiting | dark urine |
| muscle pain | difficulty breathing |
| difficult urination | loss of appetite |

Valium – is used to treat anxiety disorders:

| | |
|---|---|
| suicide thoughts | nausea |
| depressed mood | hallucinations |
| aggression | hyperactivity |

Zoloft – treats depression – panic attacks:

| | |
|---|---|
| diarrhea | fast heartbeats |
| seizures | insomnia |
| breathing that stops | impotence |

Advil – Tylenol – Pepcid – Maalox – Tums – among others – put you at risk for:

| | | |
|---|---|---|
| heart attack | kidney damage | stroke |

Medical doctors grow up with the bias that drugs are the way to go, it's how they are trained; it's imprinted in their brain in medical school, it is what they believe.

The medical profession is a service to mankind and a business for profit.

The multinational pharmaceutical drug companies are for a profit business.

Today we suffer from a host of debilitating ailments, both mental and physical, nearly all of which can be traced to the operations of the chemical and drug monopoly and which possesses the greatest threat to our continued existence.
Dr. Joseph Mercola.

What disturbs drug manufactures is that in most of their clinical trials, the placebos prove to be as effective as their engineered chemical cocktails.
Dr. Bruce Lipton.

# VACCINES

All vaccines compromise natural immunity.

Not only is vaccine efficacy dubious, today the risk for vaccine damage has significantly increased.

In the opinion of many Doctors, Scientists, and Researchers, the medical propaganda about vaccines is mostly unscientific and in many causes fraudulent.

Vaccines contain toxic ingredients that have not been adequately evaluated for long term adverse effects on humans and especially on babies and children.

The biological mechanisms for vaccine induced brain and immune dysfunction and vaccine induced immunity have not been scientifically established.

Most vaccine studies alleging that vaccines carry few risks are methodologically flawed and funded by big pharmaceutical companies or government.

Vaccines of children are considered the worst crime in the history of mankind.

It is estimated that over 1000 babies, in America alone, die from DPT vaccines every year and over 12,000 are permanently damaged.

Approximately 20% of children suffer from a "development disability" as a result of vaccines every year.

Evidence shows that immunization causes a large number of chronic diseases and death including:

| | |
|---|---|
| cancer | stroke |
| asthma | tumors |
| obesity | brain inflammation |
| diabetes | autoimmune diseases |

Vaccines are not beneficial except perhaps in a few rare instances; they do however benefit those who make and sell them.

Contrary to popular belief, avoiding vaccines is not a sign of ignorance.

Take away the profit made from vaccines and vaccines would disappear.

Ingredients in vaccines can include:

| | |
|---|---|
| glycerol | dog kidney |
| duck egg | rabbit brain |
| pig blood | antifreeze |
| chicken egg | horse blood |
| chicken embryo | aborted fetal tissue |
| human diploid cells | monkey kidney cells |
| bovine calf serum | monosodium glutamate |
| mercury thimerosal | pancreatic pig porcine |

# VACCINE WEB SITES

National Vaccine Information Center www.nvic.org

Vaccine Safety www.vaccines.net

Dr. Joseph Mercola www.mercola.com

Vaccine Liberation Organization www.vaclib.org

Precious Health Campaign http://childshoots.com

Global Vaccine Institute www.thinktwice.com

Vaccine Injured Children www.vacinfo.org

Vaccination Debate www.vacinationdebate.com

Gary Matsumoto www.without-consent.com

Canada Vaccine Risk Awareness Group www.vran.org

# 4 BLOOD TYPES – 4 DIETS

There is no perfect nutritional diet for everyone.

This explains why some people do well on vegetarian diets and others do not and also why others do well on high protein flesh food diets and others do not.

Blood Type - A - 42% population.

Vegetarian.

High carbohydrate, low fat.

Gentle exercise - yoga, swimming and golf.

Meditate - to deal with stress.

Risk factor - heart disease, cancer.


Blood Type - B – 9% population.

Varied diet - flesh foods, dairy, vegetables, fruits, nuts.

Moderate exercise – walking, biking and hiking.

Creativity – best response to stress.

Risk factor – viruses affecting immune system.

Blood Type – AB – 3% population.

Modern rare blood type.

Merging qualities of both A and B.

Calming exercise – tai chi, yoga, dance and walking.

Spirituality - best response to stress.

Risk factor - sensitive digestive system.


Blood Type – O – 46% population.

High protein diet.

Flesh foods - beef, buffalo, lamb, chicken, turkey and seafood.

Vigorous exercise – team sports, martial arts and cycling.

Intense physical exercise – best stress relief.

Risk factor – ulcers, arthritis and inflammatory diseases.

Risk factor – eating foods outside your blood type.


Eat Right 4 Your Blood Type

Dr. Peter J. D'Adamo

# STRESS

Stress – a mental, emotional or physical strain or tension.

Long term stress directly impacts:

cancer
arthritis
migraines
alzheimers
depression
inflammation

insomnia
heart disease
peptic ulcers
colds and flu's
chronic fatigue
high blood pressure

Types of Stress:

Eustress – common in athletes and executives – active – positive – strength – motivated.

Distress – is re-adjustment to situations – acute short term – chronic long term.

Hyper-Stress – pushed - overworked – overloaded.

Hypo-Stress – bored – unchallenged – restless.

Digestive and Pancreatic Stress – caused by overeating – poor diet and lifestyle.

Dehydrated Stress – very common where the body is not properly hydrated with water.

Physical Stress – involving or characterized by vigorous physical bodily activity.

Oxidative Stress – is an excess of free radicals inadequately neutralized by antioxidants.

Most people experience and suffer from multiple types of stress.

Symptoms of Stress:

| | |
|---|---|
| anger | burn out |
| diarrhea | irritability |
| sweating | constipation |
| depression | health issues |

Stress Management – tools for maintaining emotional and mental equilibrium:

| | |
|---|---|
| meditation | plenty of sleep |
| proper nutrition | hobbies – sports |
| reduce stressors | physical excercise |
| time management | simplify possessions |

Social networks very important by balancing:

| | |
|---|---|
| family | sports |
| work | friends |
| leisure | recreation |

Major stress can increase the risk of breast cancers by 12 times.

80% of all visits to doctors may be directly related to stress.

# CHRONIC DEHYDRATION

75% to 80% of the body is water.

80% to 85% of the brain is water.

As we age, we mistake thirst pains for hunger pains, so we eat instead of drinking water.

We eat food when the body should receive water.

Dyspeptic pains of:

colitis                    gastritis
heart burn                 constipation
duodenitis

Should be treated with water intake alone.

Dyspeptic pain denotes dehydration of the body.

Dehydration causes stress and stress will cause further dehydration.

Brain cell dehydration is considered the primary cause of alzheimer's.

The brain will demand water before the heart, lungs and the rest of the body, so if you get a headache from dehydration the rest of the body will be stressed and suffering greatly.

In a dehydrated cartilage, the rate of abrasive damage is greatly increased – often resulting in hip and knee replacements.

The illusions that:

Pop
Coffee
Alcohol

Manufactured Juices – are a desirable substitute for natural water needs of the body is a catastrophic mistake.

Chronic and persistently increasing dehydration is the root cause of many currently encountered major diseases of the human body.

Chronic cellular dehydration painfully and prematurely kills and body cells die, its initial outward manifestations have until now have been labeled as disease of unknown origin.

The medical profession have traditionally resorted to using drugs, medications and procedures to deal with chronic dehydration of the body.

Drink water ½ hour before meals and water 1 hour after eating but never with meals.

Drinking water with meals dilutes the natural digestive acids and enzymes creating digestive stress.

Your body needs a minimum of 6 to 8 – 8 oz. of water daily.

Water cures – don't threat thirst with medications.

# GENETICALLY MODIFIED ORGANISMS

GMO - often referred to as:

Franken foods.
Genetically engineered food.
PNT's - Plants with Novel Traits.

GMO – is as biotechnological process in which the traits and characteristics of an organism are changed by transferring individual genes from one species to another and are often referred to as genetic pollution.

GMO crops provide a significant threat to our subtle world eco system.

When humans digest genetically modified foods, the artificially modified created genes transfer into and alter the character of the beneficial bacteria in the intestines.

Between 60% - 75% of all non-organic super market processed foods tested positive for genetically modified organism ingredient contamination.

Foods that can be contaminated with GMO:

| | |
|---|---|
| soups | cereals |
| soy foods | baby foods |
| energy bars | corn syrup |
| snack foods | frozen pizza |
| frozen dinners | salad dressings |
| processed foods | meat alternatives |

GMOs approved for environmental release, food and livestock feed use:

| | |
|---|---|
| soy beans | canola |
| sugar beet | wheat |
| corn | potatoes |
| lentils | tomatoes |
| rice | squash |
| cotton | sunflower |

Health problems associated with GMO foods:

| | |
|---|---|
| diarrhea | dizziness |
| inflammation | respiratory |
| fever | viral infections |
| sterility | headaches |
| allergies | |

GMO crops – contain a special gene added that allows them to produce an insecticide.

When bugs attempt to eat the crop they are killed right away because the plant contains an invisible, built in pesticide shield.

The problem is, that when you eat this food you eat the built- in pesticide as well and this is problematic for human health and the environment.

Bio-Tech companies creating genetically modified organisms:

| | |
|---|---|
| Monsanto – USA | Syngenta – Swiss |
| Dupont – USA | BASF – Germany |
| Dow Chemical – USA | Bayer – Germany |

Countries producing genetically modified organisms:

74% - United States         10% - Canada
15% - Argentina             1% - China, Australia, South Africa


90% of world consumers demand mandatory labelling of genetically modified foods, mainly so they can avoid buying them.


Laboratory mice avoided eating genetically modified foods when given a choice.

Jeffery M. Smith

"Seeds of Deception."

www.seedsofdeception.com

# GLYCEMIC INDEX of FOODS

Glycemic index measures how fast and how much food raises blood glucose levels.

Food with higher index values raise blood sugar more rapidly than foods with a lower glycemic index values do.

Low glycemic food benefits:

| curbs appetite | slows down aging |
| encourages weight loss | staves off heart disease |
| prevents type 2 diabetes | lowers the risk of arthritis |

0 to 54:

| seeds | 0 | cauliflower | 15 |
|---|---|---|---|
| nuts | 0 | broccoli | 15 |
| cherries | 5 | cucumbers | 15 |
| eggs | 10 | peppers | 15 |
| cabbage | 10 | onions | 15 |
| beef | 12 | spinach | 15 |
| fish | 12 | squash | 15 |
| poultry | 12 | zucchini | 15 |
| tomatoes | 20 | apple | 35 |
| grapefruit | 20 | blueberries | 35 |
| raspberries | 20 | oranges | 40 |
| strawberries | 30 | grapes | 40 |
| peach | 30 | banana | 45 |
| pear | 30 | carrots | 45 |

Medium glycemic foods benefits:

| | |
|---|---|
| curbs appetite | keeps blood sugar from spiking |
| encourages weight loss | lowers the risk of disease |

55 to 69:

| | | | |
|---|---|---|---|
| corn | 55 | pineapple | 65 |
| rye bread | 60 | beets | 65 |
| brown rice | 60 | oatmeal | 65 |
| raisons | 60 | life cereal | 65 |
| bee pollen | 63 | spaghetti | 65 |
| cantaloupe | 65 | pastas | 65 |

High glycemic foods contribute to:

| | |
|---|---|
| obesity | diabetes |
| hypoglycemia | high cholesterol |
| chronic illnesses | high blood pressure |
| heart disease – cancer | exacerbate inflammation |

70 to 100:

| | | | |
|---|---|---|---|
| white rice | 70 | cherrios | 75 |
| brown bread | 70 | bran flakes | 75 |
| cream wheat | 70 | french fries | 75 |
| shredded wheat | 70 | boiled potato | 75 |
| watermelon | 75 | potato chips | 75 |
| white bread | 80 | instant rice | 90 |
| corn flakes | 85 | hard liquor | 95 |
| baked potato | 85 | sugar | 99 |
| instant potato | 85 | candy | 100 |
| honey | 87 | fructose | 100 |

# EXCITOTOXINS

Excitotoxins alter food to enhance the taste but over stimulate the brain's neurotransmitters glutamate causing brain cell death.

Excitotoxins are acidic amino acids that react with specialized receptors in the brain in such a way as to lead to destruction of certain types of neurons causing brain damage.

Higher concentrations trigger stimulation of neurons and they become very excited, firing its impulses repetitively until the point of death, hence the name excitotoxin.

List of excitotoxins:

| | |
|---|---|
| aspartame – equal | spices |
| monosodium glutamate | gelatin |
| natural beef flavouring | yeast extract |
| natural chicken flavouring | seasoning |
| hydrolized plant proteins | malt extracts |
| calcium and sodium caseinate | autolyzed yeast |
| hydrolized vegetable proteins | malt flavoring |

Excitotoxins leading to neurological disorders include:

| | |
|---|---|
| als – lou gehrigs | seizures |
| endocrine disorders | migraines |
| huntingtons chorea | alzheimers |
| hyperactivity disorder | multiple scherosis |
| attention deficit disorder | dementia complex |

Glutamate is essential for short-term and long-term memory, but problems occur when too much neurotoxins are added to our food.

Dr. Russell Blaylock

"The Taste That Kills"

www.russellblaylockmd.com

# HEPATOTOXINS

Hepatotoxins are toxic substances that damage the liver.

The liver plays a vital role transforming and clearing chemicals and is susceptible to the toxicity from drug induced agents.

Hepatotoxins include:

| | |
|---|---|
| alcohol | chlorinated solvents |
| chemicals | 900 plus medical drugs |
| heavy metals | high fructose corn syrup |

Alcohol is a hepatotoxin that alters mitochondrial and microsomal function causing fatty liver disease.

Herbicides, pesticides, industrial solvents & synthetic chemicals are hepatotoxins and contribute to major liver disease.

High Fructose Corn Syrup is a hepatotoxin, its major damage site being the liver.

More than 900 drugs have been implicated in causing liver injury and it is the most common reason for a drug to be withdrawn from the market.

Hepatotoxin drug induced liver injury is responsible for 5% of all hospital admissions and 50% of all acute liver failures.

Certain medicinal agents, when taken in overdoses and sometimes even when taken within therapeutic ranges, may injure the liver organ.

# MICRO-WAVE OVENS

Reason's to throw out your micro wave oven:

Minerals, vitamins and nutrients of all micro-waved food is reduced or altered so the body gets little or no benefit.

The human body cannot metabolize ( brake down ) the unknown by-products created by micro-wave ovens.

Male and female hormone production is shut down - or altered by continually eating ( micro-wave ) foods.

Eating ( micro-wave ) food causes loss of memory, emotional instability, concentration and a decrease in intelligence.

The minerals in vegetables are altered into cancerous free radicals when cooked in ( micro-wave ) ovens.

Micro waved foods cause stomach and intestinal cancerous growth tumors which explains the increase in colon cancer.

The prolonged eating of ( micro wave ) foods causes cancerous cells to increase in human blood.

Continual ingestion of ( micro-wave ) food causes immune system deficiencies through lymph gland and blood alterations.

Continual eating food from ( micro-wave ) ovens causes long term, permanent brain damage by shorting out electrical impulses in the brain tissue.

# ORGANIC

Organic foods are labelled organic when it has been:

grown          raised          harvested       packaged

Without synthetic chemical such as:

preservatives   pesticides      insecticides    fertilizers

Organic foods are labelled organic when not grown with Genetically Modified Plants.

When soils are used continuously the soils mineral nutrients become depleted.

Conventional farmers are then forced to saturate crops with unnatural chemical fertilizers.

Fertilizers are made up primarily of three nutrients:

nitrogen        potassium       phosphorus

Missing are the rest of the 52 minerals needed for soil health.

The quality of food depends on the quality of the soil in which the food is grown.

Organic Farming – the soil is the foundation of the food chain.

Supporting organic and sustainable agriculture is critically important to our future health and wellness.

Organic Farming production systems replenish and help maintain soil fertility, while enhancing biodiversity that protect the air, water and soil.

Organic Livestock are raised without:

| | |
|---|---|
| drugs | antibiotics |
| grains | grass fed |
| gmo foods | growth hormones |

Organic livestock farms - provide animals with "natural" living conditions and feed.

Organic livestock - health and food quality are pursued in a holistic, fresh air, exercise and good grazing approach where crowding is avoided.

When we choose organic we look after the health of our:

| | |
|---|---|
| bodies | family health |
| soil health | planet health |

Organic foods have a much higher percentage of nutrients.

# ALKALINE and ACID FOODS

PH – part per hydrogen - is a scale of 0 to 14.

Numbers below 7 are acidic – low in oxygen.

Numbers above 7 are alkaline – high in oxygen.

7.35 to 7.45 alkaline is the ideal ph for a healthy physical body.

Acid or Alkaline forming foods means the ph condition the food causes in the body after being digested.

An acidic body is a recipe for sickness, disease and aging.

Acidosis, or over-acidity of the body tissues, is one of the main causes of many arthritic and rheumatic diseases.

Eating more alkaline foods helps neutralize your body's ph oxygenating your system.

It is vitally important that there is a proper ratio between acid and alkaline foods in your diet.

The ratio in a normal healthy body is approximately 70% to 80% alkaline producing foods to 20% to 30% acidic producing.

When such an ideal ratio is maintained, the body is healthy and has a strong resistance against disease.

Acidifying Animal Protein:

| beef | pork | turkey | shell fish |
| chicken | fish | lamb | organ meats |

Acidifying Vegetables and Fruits:

| | | |
|---|---|---|
| soybeans | red beans | blueberries |
| green peas | canned fruits | plums |
| winter squash | olives | lentils |

Acidifying Grains and Nuts:

| | | | |
|---|---|---|---|
| rye | barley | oats | pecans |
| spelt | corn | rice | peanuts |
| wheat | kamut | cashews | walnuts |

Acidifying Fats and Oils:

| | | |
|---|---|---|
| butter | canola oil | olive oil |
| cheese | hemp oil | sun flower oil |
| corn oil | flax oil | sesame seed oil |

Acidifying Other:

| | | |
|---|---|---|
| sugar | wine | aspirin |
| corn syrup | hard alcohol | drugs |
| beer | coffee – tea | soft drinks - pop |

Alkalizing Vegetables:

| | | | |
|---|---|---|---|
| beets | chlorella | green beans | pumpkin |
| broccoli | cucumber | green peas | radishes |
| carrot | cauliflower | lettuce | spinach |
| celery | eggplant | onions | tomatoes |
| cabbage | garlic | sweet potato | peppers |

Alkalizing Fruits:

| | | | |
|---|---|---|---|
| apple | cherries | lemon | peach |
| avocado | cantaloupe | melon | pear |
| banana | grapes | nectarine | raspberry |
| blackberries | grapefruit | orange | strawberry |

Alkalizing Other:

| | | |
|---|---|---|
| coconuts | coconut milk | coconut oil |

# PROCESSED and FAST FOODS

90% of food budgets are spent on processed, refined and fast foods.

Processed - Refined - Fast Foods – do not serve the body.

These foods are and can include:

| | |
|---|---|
| pesticides | growth hormones |
| antibiotics | artificial coloring |
| de-natured | loaded with sugar |
| preservatives | genetically modified |
| trans fats | monosodium glutamate |
| excitotoxins | high fructose corn syrup |
| chemical laden | bottled – canned - boxed |

Processed – Refined – Fast Foods are:

depleted of vital nutrients.
leads to under nourishment.
disrupts our biological terrain.
causes fatigue and weight gain.
accelerates intestinal rotting and composting.

These foods contain insignificant:

| | | |
|---|---|---|
| minerals | proteins | vitamins |
| nutrients | fats | |

# SOY

Soybeans are mostly genetically modified.

Soy has the highest percentage of pesticide contamination.

Soy is found in:

| | | |
|---|---|---|
| soups | diet foods | meat substitutes |
| beverages | baby foods | processed foods |

Soy Baby Formulas - the worst choice for infants containing an equivalent of 4 to 5 birth control pills worth of estrogen daily.

Most soy baby formulas have 80 times the amount of manganese as breast milk and can cause brain dysfunction

Soy milk can cause:

| | |
|---|---|
| asthma | allergies |
| thyroid problems | gastro intestinal damage |

Soy contains Hemagglutinin, a clot promoting substance so blood cells cannot properly absorb oxygen, creating cardiac ill health.

Soy contains a potent enzyme-inhibitor Trypsin blocking protein digestion and may cause pancreatic disorders and stunted growth.

High levels of Phylic Acid in soy reduces assimilation of calcium, magnesium, copper, iron, zinc and vitamin D all needed for healthy bones.

Soy Phytoestrogens disrupt endocrine function and have the potential to cause infertility and breast cancer in women.

Soy Phytoestrogens are potent anti-thyroid agents that cause hypothyroidism and can cause thyroid cancer, constipation, fatigue, lethargy and weight gain.

Vitamin B12 analogs in soy are not absorbed and actually increase the body's requirement for B12.

Health problems associated with soy:

| | | |
|---|---|---|
| fatigue | kidney stones | pregnancy disorders |
| lethargy | stunted growth | infant abnormalities |
| infertility | cardiac health | pancreatic disorders |
| weight gain | constipation | severe food allergies |
| breast cancer | brain damage | pancreatic disorders |

Soy products listed below are fermented, which neutralize the phylic acid and are recommended fermented soy products.

Temph - a soybean cake with nutty, mushroom like flavour.

Miso - soybean paste commonly used in miso soups.

Natto - soybean with a sticky, strong cheese like flavour.

Soy sauce - traditionally made from fermenting soybeans, salt and enzymes.

Tofu – is not fermented and not recommended as a food.

Dr. Kaayla Daniel

The Whole Soy Story

www.naughtynutritionist.com

The Weston A. Price Foundation

# SALT – ESSENCE of LIFE

Table Salt:

After processing ordinary refined table salt at 1200 F most of the minerals have been removed except sodium and chloride.

The salt crystals are totally isolated, separated, dead and totally useless.

In order for the body to metabolize these crystal salts, it must sacrifice a tremendous amount of energy resulting in a damaging loss and zero gain.

Sea Salt:

Produced by evaporation of sea water with little processing.

Sea Salt content of the oceans is similar to the salt content of our human blood.

The mineral content gives it a different color and taste than table salt.

Sea Salt has a rich mineral content giving it a great taste.

Depending on the region salts come from, they can vary greatly in color and mineral content.

Due to the pollution of oceans, the crystalline structures may be separated making them more difficult to be absorbed.

Gord Lund

Himalayan Crystal Salt:

100% pure and the most beneficial containing 84 minerals.

The crystal is not isolated from the inherent mineral content of 84, but is connected to them in a harmonious state giving the salt a great taste.

The energy content in the form of mineral's, is balanced and can be easily metabolized by the body.

The crystal is full of life and when taken as food, will have a vital energetic effect on the body resulting in a positive gain.

Benefits - of unrefined natural salts biological process:

blood plasma
amniotic fluid
lymphatic fluid
extracellular fluid
caring nutrients in and out of the cells
sending communications to the muscles
regulating propagation to the nerve cells
lining blood vessels regulating blood pressure

# PASTEURIZED MILK
# RAW MILK

After pasteurization milk becomes acid producing in the body.

Pasteurization of milk creates a dead, white liquid that is not beneficial to your health.

Milk Pasteurization:

destroys proteins
destroys lactoferrins
destroys immunoglobulins
minerals completely unusable
destroys anti-microbial peptides
fats are damaged and destabilized
vitamins rendered biologically unusable
enzymes are denatured and less digestible

Milk pasteurization contributes to:

| | | |
|---|---|---|
| arthritis | heart disease | crohns disease |
| leukemia | osteoporosis | colic in infants |
| colon cancer | breast cancer | promotes pathogens |

Milk has to be pasteurized, because it is often loaded with non-beneficial bacteria.

Milk cows are confined and routinely given antibiotics to counter ill health, immune issues, questionable living conditions and mastitis, creating pus and blood in the milk.

A single glass of pasteurized milk can contain a mixture of as many as 20 different:

antibiotics                    growth hormones r.bgh
pain killers                   high content of pus and blood


Organic raw milk - comes from:

grass fed cows                 cows living in healthy environments


Cows not infected with:

antibiotics                    growth hormones


Benefits of organic raw milk:

healthful food                 beneficial amino acids
beneficial raw fats            rich in conjugated linoleic acid
bio available proteins         vitamins a b c d e and k


balanced blend of minerals, calcium, magnesium and iron

60 digestive enzymes and immunoglobulin antibodies

# ALCOHOL

Alcohol creates a deficiency of gamma amino butyric acid resulting in symptoms of:

| | | |
|---|---|---|
| insecurity | cravings | panic attacks |
| fearfulness | insomnia | free floating anxiety |

Candida Albicans - love to grow in alcohol.

Cirrhosis of the Liver - occurs when damaged liver cells are replaced by scar tissue.

Anemia - decrease in red blood cells and hemoglobin becomes less than normal.

Psychosis - when the ability to relate to other people and their environment is impaired.

Cardiomyopathy - disorder affecting the heart muscle cells resulting in the heart being unable to pump blood effectively.

Polyneuropathy - nerves throughout the body malfunction simultaneously, affecting senses and movements.

Alcohol Gastritis – is inflammation of the stomach caused by viruses, bacteria and an excess consumption of alcohol.

Alcohol Dementia - common and potentially severe consequences of long-term heavy alcohol consumption.

Chronic Pancreatitis - long standing inflammation altering normal structure and function of the pancreas.

Mal-absorption – an abnormality in the absorption of food leading to mal-nutrition.

Cancer - alcohol increases the risk of:

| | |
|---|---|
| liver cancer | colon cancer |
| brain cancer | rectum cancer |
| breast cancer | ovarian cancer |
| prostate cancer | stomach cancer |

Fetal alcohol spectrum disorder - alcohol during pregnancy:

| | |
|---|---|
| abortion | premature birth |
| withdrawal | facial deformities |
| slow fetal growth | mental retardation |

Alcohol - suppresses the production of melatonin which is essential for restful sleep.

# SUGAR

Sugar can and does destroy your health.

We consume an average of 145 lbs of sugar per person, per year, creating a metabolic disorder known as hypoglycemia.

Sugar has:

No minerals
No vitamins
No enzymes
No amino acids assisting digestion and absorption of nutrients.

When sugar is constantly overused, the pancreas eventually wears out and is no longer able to clear sugar from the blood, and diabetes is often the result.

Sugar increases the urinary output of vitamins and minerals.

Sugar increases the overgrowth of candida yeast organisms.

List of results of excessive sugar consumption:

| | | |
|---|---|---|
| obesity | asthma | weak eyes |
| arthritis | free radicals | indigestion |
| eczema | gum disease | appendicitis |
| allergies | feeds cancer | osteoporosis |
| gall stones | heart disease | hemorrhoids |
| weight gain | tissue elasticity | oxidative stress |
| depression | blood pressure | ulcerative colitis |
| tooth decay | premature aging | multiple sclerosis |

Sugar corrupts muscle performance and impedes strength.

Sugar turns into fat and destroys your health.

Healthy sugar alternatives:

Coconut palm sugar:
Low glycemic index of 35.
Harvest from the nectar of coconut palm trees.


Stevia:

Zero calories.

Zero glycemic index.

Plant derived.

Healthy sweetener.

20 times sweeter than sugar.


www.energyfiend.com

# POP – SOFT DRINKS

We drink an average of 56 gallons of soft drinks per year.

One can of pop contains an average of 10 teaspoons of sugar.

Drinking one pop a day for one year we consume about 15.6 pounds of sugar.

Pop contains:
Salt – creating thirst.
Caffeine – 12 oz. can = 34.5 mg.
Sugar or high fructose corn syrup a liver toxin.

Diet Pop contains:
Aspartame – known toxic poison.
Caffeine – 12 oz. can = 45 mg.

After drinking just one – 12 oz. can of pop.

Within 10 minutes – the only reason you don't vomit as a result of the overwhelming sweetness is because phosphoric acid cuts the flavor.

Within 20 minutes – your blood sugar spikes, and your liver responds to the resulting insulin burst by turning massive amounts of sugar into fat.

Within 40 minutes – caffeine absorption is complete; your pupils dilate, your blood pressure rises, and your liver dumps more sugar into your blood stream.

Within 45 minutes – your body increases dopamine production which stimulates the pleasure centers of your brain – physically identical response to heroin.

Within 60 minutes – you'll start to have a sugar crash.

One pop per day increases your risk of diabetes by 85%.

The over consumption of sweet drinks and pop is one of the leading causes fueling the world-wide obesity epidemic.

www.energyfiend.com

# ARTIFICAL SWEETNERS

Aspartame – Nutra Sweet – Equal – Amino Sweet.

Are all identical products.

Made from genetically modified bacteria using amino acids.

Addictive.

Excitotoxin.

Genetically engineered carcinogen.

Found in 6000 products to include:

| | |
|---|---|
| cereals | maple syrup |
| juice drinks | instant ice tea |
| jams and jellies | pies sugar free |
| chewing gum | gelatin sugar free |
| nutritional bars | cookies sugar free |
| processed foods | meal replacements |
| yogurt sugar free | carbonated soft drinks |
| ice cream sugar free | protein nutritional drinks |

Possible Side Effects:

| | | |
|---|---|---|
| migraines | vision | cancer |
| depression | tumors | seizures |
| heart racing | nausea | join pain |
| memory loss | headaches | mood swings |

Neotame:

May actually be an even more potent and dangerous neurotoxin, immune toxin and excitotoxin, than aspartame.

Neotame – is like aspartame on steroids and more toxic.

Neotame – called Sweetos in cattle feed and used to mask the unpleasant taste and odor improving the palatability.

Avoid Neotame at all costs if you care about your health.


Sucrose and Splenda:

Sugar derivative chemical found in the following products:

| soups | fast foods | cereals |
|-------|-----------|---------|
| juices | ethnic foods | baby foods |
| breads | sports drinks | canned fruits |
| candies | luncheon meat | canned vegetables |


Sucrose and Splenda – possible side effects:

| cancer | anemia | enlarged brain |
|--------|--------|----------------|
| diabetes | obesity | food intolerance |
| cataracts | allergies | enlarged kidney |
| heart disease | enlarged liver | enlarged colon |


Xylitol – sugar alcohol with minor digestive issues.

Sorbitol – genetically modified sugar alcohol – clinical use.

Mannitol – genetically modified sugar alcohol – clinical use.

Dextrose – commercial form of glucose – produced from starch synthetically.

Agave – 59% to 67% fructose – is heated – fractionated – non enzymatic.

Glucose – natural to the body – energy of life – comes naturally from fruits with fibre.

Artificial sweeteners – have no place in a healthy diet.

Dr. Joseph Mercola

"Sweet Deception"

# HIGH FRUCTOSE CONSUMPTION

We dangerously consume approximately 135 grams of fructose per person, per day.

To maintain optimum health keep fructose consumption under an average of 25 grams per day.

| medium   | prune        | 1.2  |
|----------|--------------|------|
| medium   | apricot      | 1.3  |
| one cup  | raspberries  | 3.0  |
| medium   | kiwi fruit   | 3.4  |
| one cup  | blackberries | 3.5  |
| one cup  | cherries     | 4.0  |
| one half | grapefruit   | 4.3  |
| medium   | nectarine    | 5.4  |
| medium   | peach        | 5.9  |
| medium   | orange       | 6.1  |
| medium   | banana       | 7.1  |
| one cup  | grapes       | 12.4 |

Fruits contain fructose, although an ameliorating factor is that whole fruits also contain vitamins and other antioxidants that reduce the hazardous effects of fructose.

Consuming excessive amounts of fructose primarily in the form of high fructose corn syrup is the fastest way to destroy your health.

Refined juices are nearly as detrimental as soda, because a glass of processed pasteurized juice is loaded with fructose, and most antioxidants are lost in the processing.

Pancreatic tumor cells use fructose to divide and proliferate.

High fructose consumption causes blood pressure to skyrocket.

High fructose consumption drives up uric acid levels possibly creating gout, the crystallization of uric acid in the joints.

High Fructose consumption packs on weight faster than any other nutrient.

Excessive Fructose consumption speeds up cancer growth.

Restricting fructose consumption is a crucial part of a cancer treatment plan.

High fructose – in its many disguises, is conveniently and deceptively called:

| | | |
|---|---|---|
| inulin | agave syrup | iso glucose |
| chicory | tapioca syrup | dahlia syrup |
| fruit fructose | glucose fructose syrup | crystalline fructose |

# HIGH FRUCTOSE CORN SYRUP

Corn is not a vegetable but a grain.

High fructose corn syrup is made from cornstarch.

High fructose corn syrup has:

not vitamins
no minerals
no enzymes
no antioxidants

Eating whole fruits does not cause the same problems as high fructose corn syrup, because fruits contain:

vitamins
minerals
enzymes
antioxidants
metabolizing the fructose.

High fructose corn syrup does not suppress the hunger hormone, so people tend to over eat.

High fructose corn syrup is a liver toxin – metabolized the same way as alcohol.

High fructose corn syrup has an extremely high glycemic index of 95 to 100.

High fructose corn syrup is 100% processed in the liver producing body fat.

High fructose corn syrup can contribute to:

| | |
|---|---|
| depression | inflammation |
| premature aging | hypertension |
| cancer – obesity | diabetes type 2 |
| chronic kidney disease | chronic fatigue |
| cardiovascular disease | raising uric acid – gout |
| fibrosis – liver scaring | overgrowth of candida yeast |

High fructose corn syrup is found in:

| | | | |
|---|---|---|---|
| gum | jams | jellies | cookies |
| soft drinks | fruit juices | diet foods | candy bars |
| dairy foods | canned foods | baked foods | processed |

High fructose corn syrup is so cheap it is added to virtually every processed food.

# ANTIBIOTICS

An antibiotic is given for the treatment of an infection caused by bacteria.

Antibiotics are not effective against viruses.

Antibiotic overuse is associated with detrimental effects on your gut bacteria.

Antibiotics – kill off part of the intestinal flora upsetting its balance, opening the door to infection or pathological over growth, killing both the good and bad bacteria.

Antibiotics permanently alter your gut bacteria and interfere with important hormones secreted by your stomach, leading to increased appetite and body fat.

Regions with the highest levels of antibiotic overuse also have the worst health status including the highest rates of:

| | | |
|---|---|---|
| obesity | diabetes | asthma |
| heart attack | strokes | heart disease |

Children taking antibiotics are the most common cause of emergency department visits for adverse drug events.

Antibiotics are over prescribed in modern medicine, and also over used in agriculture.

70% of antibiotics are used in animal feed.

Avoiding antibiotics in your food and using them for bacterial infections only when necessary go a long way towards protecting your health.

The more antibiotics we prescribe the more resistant the bacteria becomes.

# PROBIOTICS

A probiotic is a supplement containing live bacteria that supports normal gastrointestinal flora, given especially after depletion of flora caused by ingestion of an antibiotic drug.

Proper bacteria in your gut are essential for optimum health.

Antibiotic treatment, e-coli and acidic forming foods destroy normal intestinal bacteria.

Lack of certain gut bacteria can cause severe imbalances and overabundance of other strains of unfavorable bacteria can also cause severe metabolic disturbances.

Failure to replace friendly bacteria with probiotics causes further health problems.

Probiotics replace friendly bacteria after:

| | | |
|---|---|---|
| stress | poor diet | after taking laxatives |
| fasting | cleansing | after taking antibiotics |


Probiotics that promote small intestinal health:

lactobacillus
lactobacillus acidophilus


Probiotics that promote large intestinal health:

bifidobacterium bifidum
bafidobacterium infantis

Benefits of probiotics:

| | |
|---|---|
| reduces cholesterol | eliminates gas |
| synthesize vitamins | maintain regularity |
| control inflammation | reduce blood pressure |
| support immune system | produce digestive enzymes |
| control acid/alkaline levels | controls over all health |

Probiotics – contain actual live bacteria for the purpose of repopulating the intestinal tract with beneficial bacteria.

# FERMENTED FOODS

Fermented foods play an important role in digestive health.

Fermented foods were invented long before refrigeration.

Historically, mankind has consumed large amounts of probiotics in the form of fermented foods.

With every mouthful of fermented foods you consume trillions of beneficial bacteria.

Fermented foods not only give you a large variety of beneficial bacteria, they also give you more of them, so it's cost effective.

One serving of fermented vegetables is equal to an entire bottle of a potency probiotics.

Fermented foods include:

| | |
|---|---|
| kefir – milk | miso – beans |
| yogurt – milk | sourdough – rye |
| tempeh – beans | pickles – cucumber |
| natto – soybeans | sauerkraut - cabbage |

Reasons to eat fermented foods:

| | |
|---|---|
| rich in enzymes | preserves food |
| beneficial bacteria | potent detocifier |
| absorption on nutrients | improves digestion |
| increases vitamin content | proper bacteria balance |

# HEALTHY GUT

The digestive tract is the hub of the body, upon which every cell and organ depends.

A healthy gut better digests food and enhances the absorption of nutrients.

A healthy gut prevents allergies and eliminates toxins.

A healthy gut protects against over-growth of micro-organisms.

Enemies of friendly gut bacteria in order of detriment:

drugs – especially antibiotics

alcohol – destroys friendly bacteria and enzymes

pasteurized dairy – aids pathogens – destroys friendly bacteria

bread – coats intestines with an unnatural mucus paste

sugar – feeds pathogens – found in most processed foods

fried foods – fried in oils – hydrogenated oils

acid forming foods – maximum 20% to 30% of diet

processed foods – found in caned, packaged and boxed foods

agriculture chemicals – found in non organic foods

chlorinated water – found in tap water – kills intestinal bacteria

Physical and mental diseases originate in the digestive tract.

80% of your immune system is located in the digestive tract.

90% of your digestion takes place in the small intestine.

# INTESTINAL TOXEMIA

Intestinal toxemia is an overgrowth of putrefactive intestinal bacteria in the small and large intestine creating toxins.

Putrefactive bacteria – live on partially digested food, especially from animal protein that accumulates in the intestines.

These toxins are then absorbed into the blood stream and accumulate in our body and brain cells significantly affecting:

mental function
physical function
emotional function
spiritual function


Conditions that stimulates bacterial putrefaction and toxemia:

| | | |
|---|---|---|
| antibiotics | drugs | over eating |
| dehydration | sugar | left over foods |
| processed foods | stress | pasteurized dairy |
| enzyme depletion | alcohol | over cooked foods |
| mineral deficiency | parasite | high flesh food diet |


Intestinal toxemia causes:

| | | |
|---|---|---|
| fatigue | tumors | nausea |
| sciatica | insomnia | diarrhea |
| allergies | arthritis | gastritis |
| malnutrition | depression | headaches |
| diverticulitis | constipation | fibromyalgia |
| thyroid deficiency | cardiac stress | chronic fatigue |

The best and quickest treatments for bowl toxicity:

fasting
cleansing
probiotics
fermented foods

# CANDIDA - CANDIDIASIS

Candida - is a fungal or yeast infection usually in the colon, but found throughout the body.

Candidiasis - is a terrible yeast infection that can create over- whelming levels of toxicity, and is associated with the onset of many serious diseases.

An acidic diet causing acidosis is a nice home for candidiasis, bad bacteria overgrowth and cancer.

1/3 of North Americans have candidiasis.

Candida is a living, fungal parasite that releases very toxic waste, which can get into the bloodstream and cause various symptoms to include:

| | | |
|---|---|---|
| cancer | rashes | fatigue |
| vaginitis | asthma | bloating |
| depression | prostatis | impotence |
| chronic diarrhea | oral thrush | poor memory |
| electrolyte drain | bad breath | menstrual cramps |

Foods and conditions that contribute to candida albicans:

| | | |
|---|---|---|
| corn | sugar | aged cheeses |
| peanuts | dairy | processed foods |
| x-rays | hypoxia | high glycemic diet |
| bread | vinegar | fructose corn syrup |
| vaccines | alcohol | antibiotics |

Candida weakens the entire human body, especially the immune system.

79 different toxins are released by the metabolism and die-off of candida.

Several studies have shown that between 79% to 97% of cancer patients also have candida.

Candida is considered by scientists the leading cause of cancer.

How to avoid candida with proper lifestyle changes:

exercise without stressing the body

eat the best diet for you blood type

limit the use of antibiotic medications

get plenty of good bacteria with probiotic supplementation

use organic natural herbs

limit the use of birth control pills

eat organic meats and vegetables

avoid meats with antibiotic and growth hormones

eat cultured and fermented foods such as sauerkraut

Herbs that help balance intestinal bacteria overgrowth:

| | |
|---|---|
| pau d' arco | garlic |
| beta carotene | oregano oil |
| grapefruit seed extract | black walnut |
| cinnamon essential oil | caprylic acid – coconut oil |

There is a strong emotional component with an overgrowth of candida.

Emotional conditions that shut down the digestive process:

| | | | |
|---|---|---|---|
| fear | anger | stress | grief |
| doubt | hatred | greed | blame |
| resentment | selfishness | jealousy | criticism |

Many people who have suffered a trauma in their lives will also experience issues with yeast/candida, as well as other diseases.

Kathy Kalif

Emotional Side of Candida

www.atlanticjourneytowellness.org

Dr. Tullio Simoncini

Cancer is a Fungus

# MUCOID PLAQUE

Mucoid Plaque - is a product of unnatural acid stimulation in the colon.

Mucoid Plaque contributes significantly to over 90% of all diseases.

Gut bile should be above a ph of 8 alkaline, but most people's ph is as low as 4.5 acidic.

A low ph below 7 is acidic, caustic and irritates the intestinal wall.

In this environment, the gut wall if forced to protect itself by secreting mucin, thereby lining the gut with a protective mucus shield called mucoid plaque.

Contributors to mucoid plaque include:

| | | |
|---|---|---|
| drugs | anger | over-eating |
| alcohol | stress | acidic beverages |
| table salt | antibiotics | lack of peristalsis |
| parasites | flesh foods | pathogenic organisms |
| acidic foods | heavy metals | eating without hunger |

Most mucus producing foods include:

| | | |
|---|---|---|
| dairy | eggs | soy |
| grains | nuts | flesh foods |

Mucus producing foods tend to stimulate the digestive tract to produce more mucus.

Fruits and vegetables are virtually free of mucoid - mucus forming activity.

Sprouted grains, seeds and beans are closer to vegetables in composition, whilst retaining the protein content ( in more complex form ) and are much less mucus forming.

Autopsies show the average person carries 7 – 15 lbs of mucoid plaque.

Obese people can have an expanded colon from 4 to 6 inches in diameter.

Best and fastest ways of removing mucoid plaque:

| | |
|---|---|
| fasting | cleansing |
| alkaline diet | healthy diet |
| mild exercise | unconditional self love |
| eliminating causes | raw fruits and vegetables |
| drinking plenty of water | minimum of acid foods |

Dr. Richard Anderson

Cleanse and Purify Thyself

# COMPOSTING

Composting or fecal impaction is where the colon is full of waste matter that is:

toxic
enlarged
fermenting

Composting creates:

| | | |
|---|---|---|
| mold | fungus | yeast |
| mycotoxins | mycosis | enlarged colon |

When the composting button is pushed, people begin to compost and they begin the cycle of degeneration resulting in cancer and other degenerative diseases.

Composting of the colon is caused by:

| | |
|---|---|
| stress | fast foods |
| alcohol | over eating |
| radiation | canned foods |
| acidic foods | irradiated foods |
| processed foods | intense pollution |
| high glycemic diet | micro waved foods |
| refined white flour | heavy metal toxicity |
| high flesh food diet | genetically modified foods |

The most obvious outward sign of composting or fecal impaction is a large and protruding abdomen.

Keys too health and turning off the composting button:

| | |
|---|---|
| fasting | cleansing |
| self love | forgiveness |
| meditation | healthy diet |
| mild exercise | mental peace |
| taking probiotics | more alkaline diet |
| eliminating causes | raw fruits - vegetables |

Dr. Richard Anderson

Cleanse and Purify Thyself

# PARASITES

Parasites can live anywhere:

| | | | |
|---|---|---|---|
| lungs | liver | brain | skin |
| muscles | heart | lymph glands | prostate |

But most live in the intestinal tract.

Most common parasites include:

Pinworms – the most common parasite in children.

Tapeworms - can cause damage to nerves.

Round worms - can lay over 200,000 eggs per day.

Hook worms - can lay 10,000 eggs per day and live 14 yrs.

Ascaris worms – largest worm – can be two feet long.

Parasites and parasite eggs can be found in:

| | |
|---|---|
| filthy environments | meat – fish – poultry |
| infected dogs – cats | drinking infected water |
| foods from infected soil | swimming in infected water |
| barefoot on infected soil | unwashed fruits – vegetables |

Parasite disease symptoms:

| | | |
|---|---|---|
| anemia | fever | rashes |
| blurry vision | chills | iching |
| blood in feces | colitis | joint pain |
| abdominal pain | nausea | congestion |
| bleeding rectum | diarrhea | chronic fatigue |

Parasites as they die, give off toxins, particularly ammonia causing flu like symptoms.

Symptoms of parasite infestation mimic many other diseases, thereby avoiding accurate medical diagnosis.

Natural remedies for intestinal parasites:

| | |
|---|---|
| golden seal | worm seed |
| black walnut | golden seal |
| grapefruit seed extract | pumpkin seeds |

Best protection from parasites is a clean and healthy functioning intestinal tract.

Fasting and cleansing is the best way to develop and maintain a healthy intestinal tract and body.

# FASTING

Fasting - works by rapidly removing dead and dying cells.

Fasting - is the best and quickest treatments for bowl toxicity.

Fasting - helps erase past deleterious eating habits and serves as an opportunity to begin a dietary program and lifestyle that is more conductive to optimal health.

Fasting – has a powerful effect on the body as well as the spirit allowing the vital life force within to rebuild and recharge.

Benefits – overall mind-body organization is increased and this curative force throws off:

clears dead cells
rejuvenates health
accumulated toxins
balances body functions


Within 4 days of fasting:

depression lifts                        anxieties fade
mind becomes tranquil                   insomnia stops
concentration improves                  creative thinking expands


Autolysis - begins two to three days of fasting and is a process of the body digesting its own cells - it selectively decomposes those cells and tissue which are:

in excess         aged          dead           diseased

# CLEANSING

Cleansing the intestinal tract, liver and gallbladder, symptoms of disease and discomfort are given a chance to subside and your health regained.

How to determine if you need to cleanse:

body odor
constipation
lack of energy
flatulence – gas
antibiotic history
body malfunction

obesity
bad breath
any disease
dry, hard stools
unusual thinness
poor complexion

Constipation is a decrease in the frequency of passage of formed stools and characterized by stools that are hard and difficult to pass.

Primary cause of constipation:

drugs
lack of fibre
poor hydration

pharmaceuticals
lack of exercise
inflammatory bowels

Ways to help your body detoxify:

Herbs - cleanse and protect the liver.

Chew slowly - digestion begins in the mouth.

Exercise - sweats and breaths out toxins – benefits circulation.

Plenty of sleep – heals the body as you rest.

Transform stress – by emphasizing positive emotions.

Avoid overeating – especially after cleansing.

Good probiotics – keeps digestive tract healthy.

Drink more water – flushes out toxins in the body.

Eat plenty of fibre – to include organic fruits and vegetables.

Colon hydrotherapy and enemas can be very helpful:

| | |
|---|---|
| restores tone | removes waste |
| loosens waste | creates bowel habits |
| relaxes muscles | repositions intestines |

Benefits of cleansing:

| | |
|---|---|
| removes toxins | strengthens colon |
| purifies blood | promotes healthy skin |
| promotes heart health | enhances memory |
| improves digestion | soothes menstruation |

Bowel movements – there are no rules for bowl movements, but the general range is from 3 times a day to 3 times a week.

Less than 3 movements a week may indicate constipation.

More than 3 watery stools a day could indicate diarrhea.

Bowel movements should be soft, easy to pass, be brown or golden brown.

Stools should have a texture similar to peanut butter and have a size similar to that of a sausage.

The spectrum of what would be considered normal, and each person's regularity is going to be highly individualized.

There is no definition of a normal bowel movement.

# EXERCISE

Physical exercise - is any bodily activity that enhances or maintains physical fitness and overall health and wellness.

The importance and benefits of regular physical exercise:

| | |
|---|---|
| enhances sleep | slows down aging |
| removes toxins | improves circulation |
| move lymph fluid | lowers risk of cancer |
| improves digestion | tones nervous system |
| creates healthy skin | lowers risk of diabetes |
| enhances elimination | stimulates internal organs |
| lowers blood pressure | strengthen muscle system |
| opens energy channels | relieves stress and tension |
| lowers risk of arthritis | lowers risk of heart disease |
| powerful anti-depressant | supplies oxygen to the cells |

Exercise – reduces insulin levels and discourages telomere shortening and aging.

If we turn exercise into stress for the body we may get aerobic benefit, but too much physical stress breaks down body function.

For most people exercise too only 50% of capacity.

Outdoor walking – hiking with your head up and smiling is considered the best single exercise according to natural healers and fitness professionals.

Exercise encourages your brain to work at optimum capacity by causing nerve cells to multiply, strengthening their interconnections and protecting them from damage.

The more physically active school children are, the better they do academically.

Recommended exercises:

| | | |
|---|---|---|
| yoga | tai-chi | hiking |
| biking | dancing | walking |
| golfing | rebounding | aerobics |
| x-c skiing | alpine skiing | stretching |
| swimming | circuit training | team sports |

Sports with violence are not recommended.

Violence in sports is causing serious harm to athletes, young and old, and driving people out of those sports.

# BREATHING

Almost every disease known to mankind is worsened or improved by how well our respiration and breathing is.

90% of our body's metabolic energy comes from breathing.

80% of the oxygen goes to the brain.

Poor breathing habits of only using 10% to 20% of our lungs tends to make the body system acidic.

Hypoxia or lack of oxygen in the body tissue causes many chronic degenerative diseases in the human body.

Hypoxia or low oxygen diminishes:

| | | |
|---|---|---|
| congestion | sight | arthritis |
| nervousness | touch | depression |
| heart disease | cancer | fungal infections |
| viral infections | asthma | bacterial infections |
| candida albicans | hearing | decreases sexuality |

Proper oxygen enhances:

| | | |
|---|---|---|
| sight | youthfulness | optimism |
| vitality | immune system | anti-aging |
| senses | mental function | enthusiasm |
| sexuality | cell regeneration | metabolism |

Percentages of toxic elimination of metabolic waste:

3% - urination

8% - defecation

19% - perspiration

70% - respiration – why exercise is so vitally important.

Respiration through our lungs from walking, hiking and gentle exercise daily greatly enhances our physical and mental health.

# NUTRIENT ENERGIES

Five nutrient energies:

cosmic
sunlight
oxygen
food
geo-electromagnetic

Cosmic energy - is the life force.

Cosmic energy - exists everywhere in the cosmos or universe.

Cosmic energy - primary nutrient absorbed through our skin and crown of the head.

Abundant cosmic energy is obtained through - meditation, total silence and deep sleep.

Sunlight energy – is the least dense and absorbed through the eyes and skin.

Sunlight – primary source of energy for all surface phenomena and life on earth.

Sunlight – controls body function, health of eyes, brain, and body and keeps energy flowing, balanced and strong.

Sunlight – contains the 7 colors of the rainbow and each color has its own wave frequency with a specific positive health energy affecting our feelings and mood.

Breath – vitamin o (oxygen) major source of energy.

Oxygen - human body is about 2/3 oxygen.

Breathing oxygen – when the body has ample oxygen, it produces enough energy to optimize metabolism and eliminate accumulated toxic waste in the tissues.

Food – the tastiest and densest form of energy representing about 10% of our energy needs.

Food energy – we depend on what we eat and we become what we eat.

Over-eating – steels energy by causing digestive stress contributing too many health issues.

Geo-electromagnetic fields – enters through our feet and our direct contact with the earth, grounding and rebalancing us.

# EARTHING - GROUNDING

Earthing – is simply walking barefoot, grounding your body to the earth.

A great way to protect your heart is grounding yourself to the earth which transfers free electrons into your body.

This grounding naturally reduces your blood viscosity, thins the blood and lowers the risk of heart attack and stroke.

Asphalt, wood, and typical insulators like plastic or the soles of your shoes, will not allow electrons to pass through to the body and are not suitable for barefoot grounding.

Lack of grounding, due to widespread use of rubber or plastic shoes, contributes to the rise if many modern diseases like chronic inflammation.

When walking barefoot on the earth, free electrons from the earth transfer into your body thru the soles of your feet.

These free electrons are some of the most potent antioxidants known to man.

Electrons from the earth have a beneficial impact on cardio- vascular disease.

Electrons from the earth cause beneficial changes including:

| | |
|---|---|
| reducing pain | lowers stress |
| increases energy | promotes sleep |
| decreases inflammation | balances hormones |

Earthing – causes your blood to thin and flow easier, causing your blood pressure to drop.

Incorporating earthing into your daily life will help accelerate tissue repair and ease muscle pain due to strenuous exercise.

Ideal locations for earthing:

| | | |
|---|---|---|
| in water | close to water | forested areas |
| in nature | sandy beaches | dewy grasses |

Earthing is as fundamental as:

air
water
sunlight
food nutrients

Sit or walk with your bare feet directly on the earth.

Dr. James Oschman

Energy Medicine

# ELECTROLYTES

Electrolytes – are minerals in your blood and other body fluids that carry electrical charges called ions, that when dissolved in water maintains the body's fluid balance.

Electrolytes:

generate electricity
maintain heart beat rhythm
muscle action and contractions

brain function
balances blood ph
nerve transmissions

Electrolyte imbalances can cause:

fever
diarrhea
vomiting
dehydration
heart disease
bone disorders

kidney disease
eating disorders
muscle cramping
sleep disturbances
endocrine diseases
enzymatic reactions

Foods excellent in replacing electrolytes are:

cantaloupe      apples           bananas         watermelon
green beans     carrots          almonds         flesh foods
26% salt brine  avocados         coconut water   oranges

Tap water or spring water does not contain electrolytes.

# ENZYMES

Enzymes help:

accelerate cleansing
attain optimal weight
accelerate detoxification
assist in the digestive process


Eight primary enzymes:

Lipase - digests fats.
Protease - digests protein.
Amylase - digests carbohydrates.
Cellulase - breaks down fibre.
Sucrase - digests most sugars.
Lactase - digests milk sugar.
Maltese - converts complex sugars from grains into glucose.
Phytase – helps overall digestion, producing vitamin B.


Heating food above 116 degree F. = 46.6 degrees C renders most food
enzymes inactive.

You should get 75% of your digestive enzymes from food.

Raw foods are enzyme–rich and consuming them raw decreases the
body's burden to produce its own enzymes.

Enzyme deficiency results in poor digestion and poor nutrient
absorption creating a variety of gastrointestinal symptoms:

| | | |
|---|---|---|
| bloating | flatulence | cramping |
| constipation | heartburn | acid reflux |

Natural ways to increase enzyme levels:

eat fewer calories
chew thoroughly
increase intake of raw foods

Enzyme rich foods include:

| raw honey | kiwi | mango |
| raw dairy | grapes | flesh foods |
| coconut oil | papaya | pineapple |
| bee pollen | avocado | olive oil |

The most powerful enzyme rich foods are those that are sprouted – seeds and legumes.

Activities in your body requiring enzymes:

| healing wounds | reducing inflammation |
| energy production | slows the aging process |
| fighting infection | removing metabolic waste |
| absorption of oxygen | proper hormone regulation |
| removing toxic waste | regulating triglyceride levels |
| dissolving blood clots | supplying nutrients into cells |
| regulating cholesterol | breaking down fats in blood |

Digestive enzyme supplementation:

If you suffer from bloating, abdominal discomfort and constipation consider digestive enzyme supplements in addition to eating more raw foods.

Enzyme supplementation – should always be taken with meals.

# FIBRE FOODS

High fiber foods help you keep regular.

High fiber foods relieve constipation.

Most industrial countries intake of fibre is about 11 grams.

For optimum health you require between 25 to 38 grams daily.

Fruits fiber content listed in grams:

| | | |
|---|---|---|
| medium | apricot | 1.0 |
| medium | plum | 1.1 |
| one cup | cantaloupe | 1.3 |
| one cup | raisons | 1.6 |
| medium | peach | 2.0 |
| one half | grapefruit | 3.1 |
| medium | orange | 3.4 |
| medium | banana | 3.9 |
| one cup | blueberries | 4.2 |
| one cup | strawberries | 4.4 |
| medium | apple | 5.0 |
| medium | pear | 5.1 |
| one cup | raspberries | 6.4 |
| medium | avocado | 11.8 |

Raw vegetable fiber content listed in grams:

| | | |
|---|---|---|
| medium | tomato | 1.0 |
| stock | celery | 1.1 |
| medium | carrot | 2.6 |
| one cup | beets | 2.8 |
| one cup | bokchoy | 2.8 |
| one cup | onions | 2.9 |
| one cup | cauliflower | 3.4 |
| one cup | cabbage | 4.2 |
| one cup | broccoli | 4.5 |
| one cup | corn | 4.6 |

Cooked vegetable fiber content listed in grams.

| | | |
|---|---|---|
| one cup | peppers | 2.6 |
| one cup | green beans | 4.0 |
| one cup | spinach | 4.3 |
| medium | sweet potato | 4.9 |
| one cup | kale | 7.2 |
| one cup | lima beans | 8.6 |
| one cup | kidney beans | 11.6 |
| one cup | black beans | 13.9 |

Benefits of a high fibre intake:

| | |
|---|---|
| removes toxins | maintains healthy weight |
| lowers cholesterol | healthy bowel movements |
| lowers diabetes risk | lowers risk of colon cancer |
| decreases hemorrhoids | lowers risk of heart disease |
| normalizes blood sugar | eliminates need for laxatives |

# FRESH RAW JUICES

Raw freshly made juices provide the body with:

minerals
enzymes
trace minerals
bioactive vitamins

Minerals speed up recovery from disease by supporting the body's own healing activity and cell regeneration.

Raw juices bring an alkaline force into the body that helps to neutralize toxic acidity from which most people suffer.

These alkalizing minerals help restore the alkaline and mineral balance in the cells.

Live juices are high in enzymes, so they are classified as biogenic or high life force rejuvenating foods.

Fresh live juices are internal baths of health and youth.

Raw juices contain an unidentified factor improving the micro-electrical tension in the tissues improving the cells ability to absorb nutrients and excrete metabolic waste.

Because the fiber is removed by extraction, raw juice has a laxative, cleansing effect, which helps to rid the body of toxins.

Health experts estimate that enzymes in juices are destroyed within minutes of juicing.

The bio-electric colloidal potential of juices diminishes significantly after juicing.

It is important to drink immediately after juicing – do not store or save raw freshly made juices.

Best vegetables and fruits to juice:

| | | |
|---|---|---|
| apple | cranberries | cabbage |
| papaya | citrus fruits | beets |
| broccoli | berries | celery |
| carrots | pineapple | leafy greens |

Fruit and vegetable juices are high in antioxidants, which counteract free radicals that cause cellular damage, aging, susceptibility to cancer and other serious health issues.

Vegetable juice does not raise insulin levels like fruit – exception is beet and carrot juice.

Excessive consumption of fruit juices increases insulin levels.

6 to 8 oz. of raw fresh juice is the recommended daily amount for consumption and health.

# ORAC FOOD VALUES

ORAC - Oxygen Radical Absorption Capacity.

ORAC value is a method of measuring antioxidant capacity of biological foods in vitro.

Higher the number, greater the health benefits.

Fruit ORAC values:

| | | | |
|---|---|---|---|
| bananas | 1,000 | cherries | 3,500 |
| peaches | 2,000 | strawberries | 5,000 |
| oranges | 2,000 | raspberries | 5,000 |
| grapes | 2,000 | blackberries | 5,500 |
| avocado | 3,000 | blueberries | 6,500 |
| apples | 3,000 | plums | 7,500 |
| gogi berries | 3,500 | cranberries | 9,500 |

Vegetable ORAC values:

| | | | |
|---|---|---|---|
| spinach | 1,000 | cauliflowers | 2,500 |
| broccoli | 2,000 | cabbage | 2,500 |
| radishes | 2,000 | garlic | 5,500 |
| beets | 2,000 | artichokes | 8,000 |

Nuts ORAC values:

| | | | |
|---|---|---|---|
| pine nuts | 500 | almonds | 4,500 |
| macadamia | 1,500 | pistachios | 7,500 |
| brazil | 1,500 | hazelnuts | 9,500 |
| cashews | 2,000 | pecans | 18,000 |

Spice ORAC values:

| | | | |
|---|---|---|---|
| garlic | 6,500 | parsley | 74,000 |
| cayenne | 19,500 | sage | 120,000 |
| chili | 23,500 | tumeric | 127,000 |
| pepper | 34,000 | cinnamon | 131,500 |
| curry | 48,500 | thyme | 157,000 |
| cumin | 50,000 | rosemary | 165,000 |
| basil | 61,000 | oregano | 175,000 |
| nutmeg | 69,500 | cloves | 290,000 |

Additional ORAC values:

| | | | |
|---|---|---|---|
| breads | 1,500 | reishi | 5,000 |
| grains | 2,000 | shiitake | 7,000 |
| cereals | 2,000 | cordyceps | 12,500 |
| white wine | 1,000 | maitake | 16,000 |
| zinfandel | 2,500 | chaga | 52,500 |
| merlot | 2,500 | cocoa | 82,000 |

Most fruits: 1,000 to 2,000. Most vegetables: 500 to 2,000.

# SEVEN RAINBOW CHAKRAS

Chakra: is a vortex energy field that connects endocrine and nervous system plexus.

Each of the seven main chakras has a specific energetic nature that corresponds to a specific color, sound and mental and spiritual awareness.

Each food relates to a specific chakra in terms of energizing, healing, cleansing, building and rebalancing the glands, organs and nerve centers associated with that particular chakra.

Red Chakra - base of the spine:

| | | |
|---|---|---|
| cherries | red apples | red peppers |
| radishes | gogi berries | strawberries |
| tomatoes | raspberries | watermelon |

Orange Chakra – navel:

| | | |
|---|---|---|
| carrots | mango | apricots |
| squash | pumpkin | grapefruit |
| cantaloupe | sweet potato | oranges |

Yellow Chakra – solar plexus:

| | | |
|---|---|---|
| pears | bananas | citrus fruits |
| nectarines | yellow apples | pineapple |
| lemons | yellow peppers | peaches |

Green Chakra – heart:

| | | |
|---|---|---|
| broccoli | pepper | celery |
| cucumber | lettuce | avocado |
| green beans | zucchini | cabbage |

Blue Chakra – throat:

| | | |
|---|---|---|
| plum | saskatoon | eggplant |
| black currents | blueberries | blackberries |

Purple Chakra – third eye:

| | | |
|---|---|---|
| grapes | pomegranates | figs |
| prunes | purple cabbage | raisons |

White Gold Chakra – crown head:

| | | |
|---|---|---|
| garlic | leeks | onions |
| cauliflower | shallots | bok choy |
| golden apples | nuts - grains | mushrooms |

Eating foods by their color is like eating a particular color from the sun bringing us closer to the forces and powers of nature.

Everything has a natural system of harmonics in relationship to the primordial vibration of the cosmic energy, this includes our food.

# THREE GUNAS

Guna – qualities of consciousness related to diet.

Guna – three states of mind and lifestyle from diet.

Sattvic: purity – light – harmonious.

Rajasic: active – passion – outgoing energy.

Tamasic: dullness – inertia – discord.

Sattvic: organic – vegan – raw – no genetically modified foods.

fruits
nuts
vegetables
grains – seeds
pure water

Sattvic benefits:

health
strength
longevity
endurance
clarity

Sattvic effects:

joyful
grateful
peaceful
loving

Rajasic: cooked foods – fried foods – no gmo.

sugar
coffee
alcohol
flesh foods
cooked vegetables

Rajasic benefits:

passion
energized
competitive
executive-like

Rajasic effects:

acidity
toxicity
degenerative
dehydration

Tamasic: over-cooked – fried – refined – gmo – processed.

fast foods
canned foods
micro waved
processed foods
artificial sweeteners
over the counter drugs

Tamasic benefits:

minimal.

Tamasic effects:

disease
obesity
lethargic
hypoglycemia

The body, emotions, mind and spirit and even our hereditary expressions are significantly affected by what we eat.

# INFLAMATION

Inflammation is the first response of the immune system to infection or injury, producing pain, redness, heat, or swelling.

Inflammation can be external or internal.

In the absence of inflammation in the body, there is no way that cholesterol would accumulate in the wall of the blood vessels and cause heart disease and stroke.

Without inflammation, cholesterol would move freely throughout the body as nature intended.

Inflammation is what causes cholesterol to become trapped.

Acute inflammation: short term-process, usually appearing within a few minutes or hours and ceasing upon the removal of the injurious stimulus.

When we chronically expose the body to injury through toxins or foods the body was never designed to process, a condition occurs called chronic inflammation.

Chronic inflammation: has a slow onset and persists for weeks, months or years and is insidious and persistent.

Over time chronic inflammation creates:

| | | |
|---|---|---|
| diabetes | arthritis | cancers |
| high blood pressure | heart disease | alzheimer's |

Chronic inflammation culprits:

1. Sugar.


2. Vegetable oils:
corn oil
soybean oil
sunflower oil


3. Trans fats:
margarine
shortenings
hydrogenated oils


4. Pasteurized:
milk
juices
cheeses


5. Grain feed beef:
antibiotics
growth hormones
genetically modified feeds

6. Processed meats containing sodium nitrate:
hams
bacon
salami
sausage

7. Alcohol:
beer
wines
hard alcohol

8. Refined grains:
pastries
white rice
white flour
white bread

9. Food additives:
aspartame
sodium nitrate
food coloring
msg – monosodium glutamate

The human body cannot process foods packed in sugar and soaked in hydrogenated oils.

# CARBOHYDRATES

Recommended nutrient percentages:

Proteins 20% - 30%

Fats 25% - 35%

Carbohydrates 45% - 55%

Carbohydrates provide the body with fuel for physical activity and proper organ function.

Carbohydrates promote health by delivering vitamin, minerals, fiber and phyto nutrients.

Carbohydrates are divided into two classes:

1. simple carbohydrates
2. complex carbohydrates

Simple carbohydrates:

convert to fat                              high glycemic index
high in sugar – absorbs quickly             spikes blood sugar


List of simple carbohydrates:

| | | | |
|---|---|---|---|
| pop | sugar | white rice | pasta |
| milk | honey | instant rice | yogurt |
| jams – jellies | corn syrup | white bread | potato chips |

Complex carbohydrates:

satiating                              slow to digest
low glycemic index                     no spiking of blood sugar


List of complex carbohydrates:

pears          broccoli        celery        onions
oranges        plums           cucumber      carrots
lettuce        spinach         apples        cauliflower
cabbage        zucchini        bananas


Benefits of a complex carbohydrate, low glycemic index diet:

Scientifically demonstrated:

weight loss                            reduced blood glucose
decreased blood pressure               improved insulin sensitivity


Commonly reported:

increased energy                       sweet craving reduced
increased concentration                compulsive eating eliminated

# PROTEINS

Recommended nutrient percentages:

Proteins 20% - 30%

Fats 25% - 35%

Carbohydrates 45% - 55%

Protein - is found in muscle, bone, skin, hair and virtually every body part and tissue.

Protein - makes up the enzymes that power many chemical reactions and hemoglobin that carries oxygen in your blood.

Protein - next to water, makes up the greatest portion of our body weight.

Protein - when broken down by digestion, the result is 22 amino acids 8 of which are essential.

Amino acids – are the chemical units or "building blocks" of the body that make up proteins.

Essential amino acids – are obtained from diet.

Non-essential amino acids – the body manufactures from proper nutrition.

The body does not store amino acids, as it does fats and carbohydrates as a result it needs a daily supply of amino acids to make new protein.

Lack of protein can cause:

| | |
|---|---|
| death | heart weakening |
| infertility | decreased immunity |
| muscle loss | respiratory weakening |
| growth failure | acid/alkaline imbalance |
| nausea | fatigue |

Best sources of protein:

| | | |
|---|---|---|
| nuts | sea vegetables | broccoli |
| cabbage | leafy vegetables | cauliflower |
| spirulina | blue green algae | flesh foods |
| beans | mushrooms | chlorella |

# FATS

Recommended nutrient percentages:

Proteins 20% - 30%

Fats 25% - 35%

Carbohydrates 45% - 55%

Fats – come in three main categories:
1. saturated fats
2. trans fatty acids
3. un-saturated fats

Saturated fats:

Flesh foods – long chain saturate – more difficult to digest.

Dairy products – long chain saturate.

Coconut oil – is a medium chain saturate – easy to digest.

Trans fatty acids:

Damaging to the heart.

Man made unnatural fats created through hydrogenation of unsaturated fatty acid vegetable oils:

margarines – shortenings.

hydrogenated vegetable oils.

Un-saturated fats.

Classified into 3 categories:

Omega 3 – polyunsaturated – essential – the body can't make.
Omega 6 – polyunsaturated – essential – the body can't make.
Omega 9 – monounsaturated – non-essential – made from other fatty acids.


Omega 3 – polyunsaturated fats - found in:

fish oils          chia seeda        flaxseed oil        krill oil


Omega 6 – polyunsaturated fats – found in:

most seeds        most seed oils    most nuts          peppers


Omega 9 – monounsaturated fats – there are no essential omega 9 fatty acids.

# FLESH FOOD NUTRIENTS

| | | | |
|---|---|---|---|
| ground beef | fats 47% | protein 53% | carbs 0% |
| t-bone steak | fats 55% | protein 45% | carbs 0% |
| sirloin steak | fats 37% | protein 63% | carbs 0% |
| | | | |
| pork chops | fats 24% | protein 76% | carbs 0% |
| cured ham | fats 46% | protein 54% | carbs 0% |
| bacon | fats 71% | protein 29% | carbs 0% |
| spareribs | fats 77% | protein 23% | carbs 0% |
| | | | |
| lamb roast | fats 50% | protein 50% | carbs 0% |
| | | | |
| chicken breast | fats 20% | protein 80% | carbs 0% |
| turkey breast | fats 5% | protein 95% | carbs 0% |
| duck breast | fats 16% | protein 84% | carbs 0% |
| | | | |
| tuna | fats 20% | protein 80% | carbs 0% |
| shrimp | fats 10% | protein 90% | carbs 0% |
| lobster | fats 5% | protein 89% | carbs 6% |
| wild coho | fats 28% | protein 72% | carbs 0% |
| farmed coho | fats 42% | protein 58% | carbs 0% |
| wild sockeye | fats 46% | protein 54% | carbs 0% |
| wild halibut | fats 19% | protein 81% | carbs 0% |
| wild cod | fats 7% | protein 93% | carbs 0% |
| wild rainbow | fats 35% | protein 65% | carbs 0% |

# FRUIT NUTRIENTS

| | | | |
|---|---|---|---|
| apples | fats 3% | protein 2% | carbs 95% |
| bananas | fats 3% | protein 4% | carbs 93% |
| grapefruit | fats 2% | protein 5% | carbs 93% |
| pears | fats 2% | protein 2% | carbs 96% |
| peaches | fats 5% | protein 8% | carbs 87% |
| watermelon | fats 4% | protein 7% | carbs 89% |
| cherries | fats 3% | protein 7% | carbs 91% |
| blackberries | fats 10% | protein 11 | carbs 79% |
| blueberries | fats 5% | protein 4% | carbs 91% |
| strawberries | fats 8% | protein 7% | carbs 85% |
| cantaloupe | fats 5% | protein 8% | carbs 87% |
| grapes | fats 2% | protein 4% | carbs 94% |
| oranges | fats 2% | protein 7% | carbs 91% |
| avocado | fats 77% | protein 4% | carbs 19% |

# VEGETABLE NUTRIENTS

| | | | |
|---|---|---|---|
| kidney beans | fats 14% | protein 35% | carbs 51% |
| navy beans | fats 9% | protein 22% | carbs 69% |
| lima beans | fats 3% | protein 20% | carbs 77% |
| spinach | fats 14% | protein 30% | carbs 56% |
| garlic | fats 3% | protein 12% | carbs 85% |
| mushrooms | fats 13% | protein 37% | carbs 50% |
| carrots | fats 3% | protein 5% | carbs 92% |
| beets | fats 3% | protein 10% | carbs 87% |
| onions | fats 2% | protein 8% | carbs 90% |
| tomatoes | fats 9% | protein 12% | carbs 79% |
| celery | fats 10% | protein 17% | carbs 73% |
| cabbage | fats 4% | protein 11% | carbs 85% |
| peppers | fats 7% | protein 10% | carbs 83% |
| peas | fats 4% | protein 23% | carbs 73% |
| squash | fats 2% | protein 5% | carbs 93% |
| cucumbers | fats 6% | protein 11% | carbs 83% |
| green beans | fats 3% | protein 14% | carbs 83% |
| zucchini | fats 16% | protein 31% | carbs 53% |
| cauliflower | fats 3% | protein 19% | carbs 78% |
| broccoli | fats 9% | protein 20% | carbs 71% |
| sweet potato | fats 1% | protein 6% | carbs 93% |

# SPECIAL FOOD NUTRIENTS

| | | | |
|---|---|---|---|
| pecans | fats 87% | protein 5% | carbs 8% |
| macadamia | fats 88% | protein 4% | carbs 8% |
| almonds | fats 72% | protein 13% | carbs 15% |
| cashews | fats 66% | protein 11% | carbs 23% |
| walnuts | fats 83% | protein 8% | carbs 9% |
| sesame seeds | fats 73% | protein 11% | carbs 16% |
| hemp seeds | fats 73% | protein 25% | carbs 2% |
| | | | |
| eggs | fats 63% | protein 35% | carbs 2% |
| milk | fats 49% | protein 21% | carbs 30% |
| cheese | fats 72% | protein 26% | carbs 2% |
| honey | fats 0% | protein 0% | carbs 100% |
| coconut oil | fats 100% | protein 0% | carbs 0% |
| chlorella | fats 20% | protein 57% | carbs 23% |
| spirulina | fats 22% | protein 48% | carbs 30% |
| | | | |
| wheat | fats 16% | protein 13% | carbs 71% |
| oatmeal | fats 14% | protein 12% | carbs 74% |
| wild rice | fats 3% | protein 14% | carbs 83% |
| brown rice | fats 7% | protein 8% | carbs 85% |
| buck wheat | fats 8% | protein 13% | carbs 79% |
| brewers yeast | fats 0% | protein 55% | carbs 45% |

# BEE POLLEN - PROPOLIS
# ROYAL JELLY

Bee pollen – is the most complete food found in nature.

Bee pollen is rich in:

| | |
|---|---|
| B12 | lecithin |
| anti radiation | minerals |
| 500 enzymes | selenium |
| all amino acids | vitamin a b c e |

Bee pollen – counteracts the signs of aging and increases both mental and physical capability.

Bee propolis – protects us from bacteria and strengthens our immune system.

Bee propolis – powerful against viruses, something antibiotics cannot do.

Bee propolis – reduces colds, coughing and inflammation of the mouth, tonsils and throat.

Royal jelly – contains every nutrient necessary to support life.

Rich source of pantothenic acid also known as B5.

Combats stress – fatigue and insomnia – a vital nutrient for healthy skin and hair.

# BLUE GREEN ALGAE
# SPIRULINA - CHLORELLA

Blue green algae – is a phyto-plankton and contains virtually every nutrient.

Blue green algae – is 60% to 70% protein and a more complete amino acid profile than beef.

Blue green algae are rich in chlorophyll and have been shown to improve brain function and memory.

Blue green algae are rich in phenyletylamine a stem cell enhancer.

Chlorella – is amazing for the immune system and for reducing cholesterol.

Chlorella – prevents the hardening of the arteries, a precursor for heart attacks and stroke.

Chlorella – is 57% protein and high in B12.

Spirulina – helps in controlling blood sugar levels and cravings.

Spirulina – is a key and vital food for diabetics.

Spirulina – is 48% protein – full spectrum of assimilable minerals – high in B12.

# COCONUT WATER
# MILK – OIL

Coconut water is one of the best sources of electrolytes found in nature.

The electrolyte molecular structure of coconut water is identical to human blood plasma.

Coconut water is low in sugar, but pleasantly sweet.

Coconut water:

has five electrolytes your body needs:

| | | |
|---|---|---|
| calcium | potassium | phosphorus |
| sodium | magnesium | including love |

Coconut milk:

is a rich source of healthy fat and used often in cooking, especially in Asian cuisine.

Coconut oil is:

| | | |
|---|---|---|
| anti-viral | anti-fungal | anti-microbial |
| anti-yeast | anti-bacterial | anti-inflammatory |

Coconut oil: 48% lauric acid giving it healing properties.

Coconut oil speeds up healthy metabolism, burning calories contributing to weight loss.

# CO ENZYME Q10
# and UBIQUINOL

Co Enzyme Q10 – is recommended for people under 40.

Ubiquinol – is recommended for people over 40.

As we age your body levels of Q10 continue to diminish.

When levels of Q10 start dropping so does your health.

Co Enzyme Q10 - called the miracle nutrient.

Support the nervous system.

Keeps organs and muscle tissue elastic.

Provides boost to your immune system.

Helps reduce the signs of aging.

Produce more energy for your cells.

Strengthen the heart and the overall cardiovascular system.

Act as an antioxidant protecting you from free radical damage.

Helps maintain blood pressure levels within a normal range.

Most importantly – keeps your heart muscle elastic.

This essential nutrient should be a top priority of an age defying strategy.

# HEMP OIL

Hemp oil has not been genetically modified and is available certified organic.

Hemp oil is rich in:
linoleic acid
alpha linoleic acid


Linoleic acid – enhances the die off of cancer cells, and is proven to have a positive health effect on the human body.

Regular use of hemp oil:
immune system stimulator
effective ant-inflammatory
reduces risk of arteriosclerosis
improves p.m.s. related symptoms
reduces risk of cardiovascular disease
alleviates symptoms of rheumatoid arthritis


Hemp oil is a preventative measure and treatment for:

cancer
multiple sclerosis
schizophrenic psychosis


Hemp oil decreases elevated blood levels of LDL cholesterol.

# HIMALAYAN CRYSTAL SALTS

Himalayan crystal salts are 100% pure and the crystals are not isolated from the inherent 84 mineral elements, but connected to them in a harmonious state.

The crystal is full of life and when taken as food, it will have a vital energetic effect on the body resulting in a positive gain.

Himalayan crystal salt brine:

Balance the energy meridians of the body in 20 minutes.

To make the brine – take the crystal salts rocks and place them in a 10 oz. jar of purified water with a ratio of 1/3 salt rocks and 2/3 water = 26% salt brine within 24 hours.

Taking a teaspoon of the brine ( sole ) with 8 oz. glass of high quality water on an empty stomach each morning gives the body energy, supports the digestive tract and cleanses the body from the inside out.

The salts themselves are beneficial as a food flavoring.

The 26% sole drink beneficial for energizing the body.

www.heartfeltliving.com

www.himalayancrystalsalts.com

# LEAFY and CRUCIFEROUS VEGETABLES

Leafy green vegetables – have the highest concentrations of digestible nutrients, fat burning compounds, vitamins and minerals protecting the body.

Leafy green vegetables – contain beneficial protein, protective photo-chemicals and healthy bacteria, building cleaner muscles and tissue.

Green super foods – are rich in chlorophyll aiding in the production of hemoglobin.

Leafy cruciferous vegetables include:

| | | |
|---|---|---|
| baby spinach | spinach | kale |
| romaine lettuce | cabbage | endive |
| mustard sprouts | swiss chard | lettuce |
| dandelion greens | collard greens | chicory |

Special cruciferous vegetables include:

| | | |
|---|---|---|
| brussel sprouts | cauliflower | arugula |
| chinese broccoli | watercress | bok choy |
| broccoli | cabbage | |

Root cruciferous vegetables include:

| | | |
|---|---|---|
| turnips | daikon | carrots |
| radishes | parsnip | kohlrabi |

Cruciferous vegetables lower heart disease and cancer risks.

# MACA

Maca is a hardy root vegetable grown in the Andes mountain plateaus of Peru.

Maca is rich in:

vitamins          phytonutrients  minerals                    amino acids

Maca is a adaptogen that supports:

stress reduction          increases stamina
adrenal function          circulatory system
endocrine system          enhances immune system

A hormonal regulator supporting the endocrine system and balance the hormones.

Regulate menstruation.

Relieve menopausal symptoms.

A sexual stimulant and fertility aid for both men and women.

Increase of sexual desire and libido.

Maca:

84 minerals          aids diabetes
balances ph          supports thyroid
arthritis relief          lowers blood pressure

# MUSHROOMS

Mushrooms – provide excellent nutrition such as:

proteins          b-vitamins – especially niacin    enzymes

Mushrooms:

promotes skin health
immune boosting properties
aids in destroying cancer cells
improves outcome of chemotherapy and radiation

Mushrooms – help protect the liver, including protection from adverse effects of alcohol consumption.

Mushrooms contain an antioxidant ergothioneine unique to mushrooms.

Ergothioneine – is an unusual sulfur containing derivative of the amino acid histidine.

Histidine – has a very specific role in protecting your DNA from oxidative damage.

Most common and healthy mushrooms:

| | | |
|---|---|---|
| reishi | chaga | oyster |
| button | maitake | shiitake |
| enokitake | portabella | brown cremini |
| corhycepts | lions mane | himematsutake |

Many medicinal mushrooms are:

anti-viral      anti-tumor       anti-inflammatory
anti-fungal     anti-bacterial   pro - health

Therapeutically – it is important to use a blend of multiple mushrooms, organically grown, rather than just one type.

Button mushrooms are an excellent low calorie food, especially for diabetics.

Mushrooms can help:

slows aging            controls blood sugar
aids blood flow        athletic performance
regenerate nerves      cardiovascular health

www.medicinalmushrooms.net

# NORI – KELP – DULSE

Nori - Kelp - Dulse – are super seaweed vegetables.

10 time more calcium than milk.

8 time more calcium that beef.

Chemical composition of seaweeds is close to human blood plasma.

These sea vegetables regulate and purify our blood system.

Nori, Kelp and Dulse help alkalize our blood.

They boost weight loss and deter cellulite build up.

Nori, Kelp and Dulse's natural iodine helps to stimulate the thyroid gland.

Seaweed vegetable minerals act like electrolytes stimulating lymphatic drainage.

# SAUERKRAUT

Sauerkraut - is one of the best natural probiotics on earth.

Sauerkraut – is made through a natural process of fermentation that creates beneficial probiotic bacteria.

One serving of fermented sauerkraut is equal to an entire bottle of quality probiotics.

It is very important that the cabbage used in sauerkraut be:

| | | |
|---|---|---|
| raw | unpasteurized | free of vinegar |
| organic | no preservatives | made with love |

Benefits of eating sauerkraut include:

regulates blood sugar
high in digestive enzymes
an abundance of vitamin c
maintains acid/alkaline balance
aids in the healing of candidiasis
various beneficial lactobacilli culture – strengthen digestion

Sauerkraut is high in acetylcholine which:

| | |
|---|---|
| improves sleep | lowers blood pressure |
| regulates bowels | calms nervous system |

# TUMERIC

Tumeric – is an amazing herb very low in calories, while dense in vitamins and minerals.

Tumeric – is a powerful antioxidant.

Puts the brakes on aging and supports eye health.

Aid the skeletal and joint health.

Support cardiovascular system and healthy liver function.

Helps maintain normal cholesterol levels.

Promote healthy and radiant skin.

Improves and balances your digestive system.

Support healthy blood and circulatory system.

Promote a healthy female reproductive system.

Boost immunity protecting against free radicals.

Assist your neurological systems healthy response to stress.

Has curcuminoids that fight cancer, arthritis and alzheimers.

Is thermogenic boosting metabolism helping to burn calories.

Tumeric – in cooking – choose a pure turmeric powder rather than a curry powder – especially from a high organic source.

# ESSENTIAL OILS

Essential oils – are widely used in:

aromatherapy          topical lotions
herbal remedies       soothing baths


Essential oils – derived from distillation of:

bark          flowers          leaves          plant roots


Examples of essential oils uses:

cedar wood oil       arthritis healer
camphor oil          antiseptic
eucalyptus oil       respiratory conditions
neroli oil           insomnia – circulation
peppermint oil       nausea – travel sickness
anise oil            rheumatism – stimulant
ginger oil           rheumatism – colds – flu's
clary sage oil       throat – sinus – congestion
lavender oil         wounds – burns – soothing
orange sweet oil     stimulatory – inflammation
geranium oil         anti-depressant – balances hormones
oregano oil          anti-yeast – anti-fungal
basil oil            anti-depressant – anti-bacterial
rosemary oil         revitalizes – stimulates – relieve stress

# VITAMIN D

Vitamin D3 – is not a vitamin but a seco steroid hormone from solar radiation – the sun.

Optimizing your sun exposure and level of D3 may be one of the most important physical steps you can take in support of your long term health.

D3 deficiency contributes to:

| | |
|---|---|
| autism | infertility |
| cancer | crohns disease |
| stroke | multiple sclerosis |
| fatigue | osteoporosis |
| diabetes | osteoarthritis |
| depression | hypertension |
| heart disease | autoimmune disease |

Sunlight is your best and ideal source of D3.

Sunlight - UV light is divided into three wavelength ranges:

UV-A

UV-B ultraviolet light generates vitamin D3 in your skin.

UV-C

Have your vitamin D3 level monitored to confirm your levels are therapeutic at 50-70 ng/ml year-round.

The best place to get D3 is from your skin being exposed to UV-B in normal sunlight.

Tanning is a natural protection against sunburn; it's what your body was created to do.

Caution – avoid sunburn – implement sun exposure gradually.

Overdosing on vitamin D3 from sun exposure is highly unlikely as your body has a built-in failsafe which will shut down production when your D3 levels are healthy.

UV-B –sunshine – is not a constant and is influenced by:

Exposure time.

Clouds can block UV-B.

Latitude – the further north – the less UV-B.

Altitude – the higher up you are, the more UV-B.

Time of year – not available in winter months.

Person age – elderly have less efficiency at producing D3.

Skin pigmentation – darker skin takes longer to produce D3.

Supplementation – with D3 is very important, especially in northern latitudes.

There are two types of oral vitamin D3.

D3 – recommended                    D2 – not recommended

Avoid D2 - has been shown to be toxic at higher dose levels.

D3 - supports the following systems and body functions:

| | | | |
|---|---|---|---|
| skin | digestion | hearing | sleep |
| hair | immunity | muscles | bones |
| eyes | respiratory | athletics | heart |
| aging | reproductive | pancreas | vascular |

An estimated 95% of North Americans are D3 deficient.

# FACTORY FARMS

CAFO - Confined Animal Feeding Operations.

CAFO's are among the most:

cruel
polluting
most disease ridden animal facilities on planet earth


Factory farms use:

antibiotics
growth hormones
genetically modified feeds

Egg laying hens – are confined in small wire battery cages.

Chickens for meat – have been genetically altered to grow twice as fast and twice as large.


Fish – raised in crowded, unsanitary, excrement-laden water.

Fish farms – use agriculture chemicals:

antibiotics      parasite disinfectants    growth hormones

Beef cattle – live in feedlots in manure laden holding pens.

Feedlot cattle – are fed growth hormones, antibiotics and fed unnaturally rich diets designed to fatten them quickly.

Pigs – are raised in close confinement, unsanitary conditions creating diseases such as porcine, respiratory syndrome, swine influenza and salmonellosis.

Half of pigs that die between weaning and slaughter succumb to respiratory diseases due to poor air quality.

Dairy cow diseases include bovine leukemia, bovine immunodeficiency virus, mastitis, and johne's disease which are rampant in modern dairies.

Drinking water located near CAFO farms are often contaminated by animal waste runoff.

People living near CAFO's are exposed to odorous emissions linked to:
asthma
nausea
premature death
neurological problems
cardiovascular ailments
decreased lung function

www.farmsanctuary.org

# PERSONAL CARE PRODUCTS

Over 800 toxic and cancer causing agents have been identified in personal care products, cosmetics and baby products.

Cosmetic chemicals on your skin, are absorbed straight into your blood stream without filtering of any kind, so there is no protection against the toxins.

Women who use make-up on a daily basis can absorb up to five pounds of chemicals into their bodies each year.

Carcinogenic ingredients found in personal care products:

Acrylamide: mammary tumors and cancers.

Coal tars: asthma – fatigue - headaches - nausea.

Parabens: hormone disrupting - damages endocrine system.

Phenol carbolic acid: paralysis – convulsions - death.

Sodium laureth sulphate: premature aging – carcinogen.

Triethanolamine tea: potential of liver - kidney cancer.

Diethanolamine DEA: potential of stomach – bladder cancer.

Prolonged daily exposure, over a lifetime of toxic ingredients, many of which are left on the skin, has a cumulative negative effect on the body, mind and spirit.

Buy organic personal care products from trusted sources.

# CLUTTER and POSSESSIONS

Clutter is stuck energy.

When clutter stagnates we experience illness and struggles.

When clutter is cleared we experience life as being harmonious.

Physical clutter reflects mental clutter in your mind.

Clearing clutter releases negative energy in the mind, body, emotions and feelings.

Types of Clutter:

| | | | |
|---|---|---|---|
| toys | junk | socks | shoes |
| tapes | books | photos | clothing |
| furniture | magazines | collections | electronics |

sports equipment
things that need fixing
unproductive relationships
clutter hoarded by a partner

Letting go of possessions that have little or no significance in your life, you literally feel lighter in body, mind and spirit.

We think we own our possessions, but in truth they own us.

Do not posses anything which one does not really need, for instance, one must not keep a chair if one can do without it.

In observing this principal one is led to a progressive and positive simplification of one's own life. Mahatma Ghandi

# PEOPLE POLLUTION

Everything in the universe vibrates at all levels of vibration:

Love – vibrates at a high vibration.

Hate – vibrates at a low vibration.

People emit both positive & negative electro-magnetic energy:
positive – high vibration
negative – low vibration

Negative people leave you feeling:
drained
exhausted
uncomfortable

Positive people leave you feeling:
uplifted
peaceful
empowered

Ways to overcome negative influences:

walking in nature             energy of laughter
keeping good company          joy of radiating love
avoiding violent television   avoiding negative people

Be responsible for the energy you bring into other people's space.

# VISUAL POLLUTION

Visual image pollution – offends our eyes and impacts our overall well being.

Visual pollution is when the natural environment has been downgraded.

Examples of visual image pollution:

| | | |
|---|---|---|
| war | polluted water | garbage in streets |
| graffiti | open pit mines | violence in sports |
| city smog | clear cut forests | violence in hockey |
| power lines | urban degradation | outdoor neon signs |

murders and violence on television
violence and murders in video games

The average 14 year old will have seen approximately 14,000 violent murders on television.

What we visually see affects our:

| | |
|---|---|
| mental health – wellness | spiritual health - wellness |
| physical health -            wellness | emotional health – wellness |

A healthy visual environment promotes the values of those who live, work and play in that community; it promotes civic pride and economic health.

# THOUGHT POLLUTION

Everything in the universe was a thought first.

Causes of thought pollution:

over thinking
repeatedly analyzing
focusing and rehashing problems
continuous stream of negative thoughts
concerns and worries that plague our lives
excessive talking about our problems and issues

Problems may not be worse but thinking makes it so.

Thought pollution will cause you to become emotionally distraught.

Accepting everything that happens in your life without:

hatred         anger         resentment    bitterness

Simple solutions:

living in the present
spending time in nature
meditation – quieting the mind
reading inspirational and positive books

The only power anything has in your life is the power you give it "so"
keep good thoughts and good company.

# WORDS - THOUGHTS
# FEELINGS - ACTIONS

What we say, think, feel and do affects every person, place, condition and thing in the universe including ourselves.

Thieves of the heart:

| | | | |
|---|---|---|---|
| anger | fear | selfishness | blame |
| doubt | greed | judgement | gossip |
| hatred | self pity | resentment | jealousy |
| criticism | unworthiness | condemnation | |

Qualities of wholeness:

| | | | |
|---|---|---|---|
| love | joy | peace | purity |
| beauty | balance | respect | harmony |
| kindness | simplicity | perfection | compassion |

Three loves:

conditional love – based on meeting certain conditions – ego
unconditional love – no conditions to meet – spiritual
unconditional self love – universal panacea

Three minds:

conscious mind – reasoning mind – computer programmer
subconscious mind – non reasoning – runs body – computer
super conscious mind – all knowing – conscience - intuition

Ask yourself – is what I am thinking, and feeling in this moment what I want to empower and create in my life?

# GLOSSARY

Acidosis - a physical and mental state that occurs when the body becomes too acidic.

Alkalosis – a physical and mental state that occurs when the body becomes too alkaline.

Antioxidant – any substance that reduces the damage caused by oxidation, such as harm caused by free radicals.

Autotoxemia – a state in which the body cells begin to die due to toxic overload.

Bio-active – having an effect on or causing a reaction in living tissue.

Carcinogenic – producing or tending to produce cancer.

Colloidal – a fluid solution in which the particles are evenly distributed.

Chronic – suffering from disease or ailment of long duration or frequent recurrence.

Colitis – inflammation of the large intestine causing abdominal pain.

Duodenitis – inflammation of the upper segment of the small intestine.

Dyspeptic – denotes dehydration – pain of gastritis, duodenitis and heart burn.

Excitotoxins – foods that damage and kill nerve cells by excessive stimulation of brain neurotransmitters.

Endocrine – glands producing secretions to help control bodily metabolic activity to include pituitary, thyroid, adrenals, ovaries, and testes.

Extracellular – is fluid outside the cells – the inner ocean of the body that bathes the cells.

Free radicals – are toxins and pollutants that damage the cells, proteins and DNA accelerating disease.

Gastritis – inflammation of the stomach lining with symptoms of burning and discomfort.

Glycemic – a measure of the effects of carbohydrates on blood sugar levels.

Hepatotoxins – a poison, usually a drug or alcohol that is harmful to the liver.

Hydrogenation – hardening of fats in which liquid oils are turned into solid fats.

Hypoglycemia – an endocrine stress imbalance in which the body is not able to balance blood sugar; resulting in physical, emotional and mental problems.

Immunoglobulin – soluble proteins that are involved in the recognition, binding or adhesion process to cells.

Inflammation – reaction causing redness, warmth, swelling and pain as a result of infection, irritation or injury – inflammation can be internal or external.

Lactoferrin – derives a large portion of its unique ability to bind iron.

Iatrogenic – medical errors by medical doctors causing death.

Metabolic – a biochemical process within the cells that produces heat energy for the body.

Microorganisms – an organism of microscopic or ultra-micro- scopic size.

Mitochondria - produce energy for the cells through cellular respiration.

Mycotoxins - a poisonous substance produced by fungus, especially mold.

Ovolactovegetarian – one who eats eggs, dairy and vegetarian foods, but not flesh foods.

Pathogenic – a specific causative agent ( as bacteria or virus ) of disease.

Phenyletylamine – PEA ( molecule of joy ) a natural mood elevator and anti-depressant.

Toxemia – a condition in which the blood contains toxins produced by body cells at a local source of infection or derived from the growth of micro-organisms.

# REFERENCE BOOKS

Conscious Eating – Dr. Gabriel Cousens

Rainbow Live Green Food Cuisine – Dr. Gabriel Cousens

You Can Heal Your Life – Louise L. Hay

Your Body's Many Cries for Water – Dr. F. Batmanghelidj

Water Cures : Drugs Kill – Dr. F. Batmanghelidj

Take Control of Your Health – Dr. Joseph Mercola

Sweet Deception – Dr. Joseph Mercola

Eat Right for Your Type – Dr. Peter J. D'Adamo

Seeds of Deception – Jeffery M. Smith

The Whole Soy Storey – Dr. Kaayla Daniel

Healing With Whole Foods – Paul Pitchford

Cleanse and Purify Thyself – Dr. Richard Anderson

The Taste That Kills – Dr. Russel Blaylock

The Emotional Side of Candida – Kathy Kalaf

Energy Medicine – Dr. James Oschman

Cancer is a Fungus – Dr. Tullio Simoncini

The Biology of Belief – Dr. Bruce Lipton

# REFERENCE WEB SITES

www.mercola.com - Dr. Joseph Mercola

www.ResponsibleTechnology.org - Jeffery H. Smith

www.vitamincouncil.org - Dr. John Cannel

www.nvic.org - National Vaccine Information Center

www.vaccines.net - Vaccine Safety

www.vran.org - Canada Vaccine Risk Awareness

www.russellblaylockmd.com – Dr. Russell Blaylock

www.atlanticjourneytowellness.org – Kathy Kalif

www.vacinfo.org - Vaccine Injured Children

www.naughtynutritionist.com – Dr. Kaayla Daniels

www.wanttoknow.infodeception10pg - Genetically Modified

www.greenpeaceusa.org - Genetically Modified Foods

www.heartfeltliving.com - Himalayan Crystal Salts

www.farmsanctuary.org - Factory Farms

Univ. of California San Francisco - Dr. Robert H. Lustig

www.ingramcontent.com/pod-product-compliance
Lightning Source LLC
Chambersburg PA
CBHW020414290526
45785CB00002B/552